JEANNE JONES' FOOD LOVER'S DIET

Jeanne Jones' Food Lover's Diet

BY JEANNE JONES

Medical Preface
HAROLD RIFKIN, M.D.

Nutritional Preface
BARBARA E. GUNNING, Ph.D., R.D.

CHARLES SCRIBNER'S SONS • NEW YORK
101 PRODUCTIONS • SAN FRANCISCO

Copyright © 1982 Jeanne Jones

Library of Congress Cataloging in Publication Data

Jones, Jeanne.
　Jeanne Jones' Food lover's diet.

　Bibliography: p.
　Includes indexes.
　1. Reducing diets.　I. Title.　II. Title:
Food lover's diet.
RM222.2.J623　1982　　613.2'5　　82-12554
ISBN 0-684-17795-1

1 3 5 7 9 11 13 15 17 19　K/C　20 18 16 14 12 10 8 6 4 2

Printed in the United States of America

TO VIOLA STROUP
for helping me to turn a concept into a reality.

IN GRATEFUL ACKNOWLEDGMENT:
Eleanor Bine for manuscript material
Nancy Bohannon, M.D., for manuscript material
Barbara Chesnut, B.S. Nutrition, for data research
Barbara Gunning, Ph.D., R.D., for technical advice and assistance
Lee Ann Jones for recipe testing

Some of the recipes and charts in this book have been revised and updated from material that originally appeared in other books by Jeanne Jones, published by 101 Productions.

The target heart rate and personal heart rate charts were reprinted from *Fitness First*, copyright 1980 by Jeanne Jones and Karma Kientzler (101 Productions) with the permission of Karma Kientzler.

James Beard's recipe for overbaked potatoes has been included with the permission of James Beard. This and the recipe for stuffed baked potatoes were reprinted by permission of M. Evans and Company from *Stuffed Spuds: 100 Meals in a Potato*, copyright 1982 by Jeanne Jones.

The definition of vegetarianism was repinted from the winter 1981–1982 issue of *Vegetarian Voice*, the quarterly newspaper of the North American Vegetarian Society, with their permission.

Contents

MEDICAL PREFACE

Jeanne Jones has done it again. Her previous books attest to her basic knowledge of the concepts of nutrition, to her meticulous attention to detail and to her remarkable ability to present the facts in a realistic, intelligent, easily readable and no-nonsense approach.

The present volume, *Food Lover's Diet,* is a superb comprehensive guide for individuals who wish to lose weight, and more significantly, who wish to maintain their desired weight, once the pounds are lost.

In this volume Jeanne Jones does a masterful job of presenting the basic concepts of diet, including a thoughtful analysis of the various caloric sources and their differences. She stresses the rationale for fat and cholesterol restriction and the multifaceted problems associated with alcohol intake. The reasons for monitoring the amount of salt and refined carbohydrates in the diet are outlined in a clear, intelligent, clinically sound and concise fashion. Additionally, she reaffirms the need and importance of including fiber and complex carbohydrates in the diet. Further, it takes a special individual like Jeanne Jones to include, in this day and age, the economic advantages of her diet as well.

Her encyclopedic knowledge of healthful dieting and cooking is once again demonstrated in this volume, proving that healthy eating can be exciting and tasty and still accomplish the major purpose of losing and maintaining weight loss without ever losing one's feeling of well-being.

HAROLD RIFKIN, M.D.
Clinical Professor of Medicine
Albert Einstein College of Medicine
Principal Consultant, Diabetes Research and Training Center,
Albert Einstein College of Medicine
Montefiore Hospital and Medical Center,
New York, New York

NUTRITIONAL PREFACE

Food Lover's Diet provides an exciting, sound and intelligent compilation of nutritional data that can be used effectively by the novice as well as the professional nutritionist.

Currently, it is popular to "think thin." This concept has evolved from the merging of two ends of the body beautiful spectrum, which includes a growing concern with health as well as body appearance. Many of the current weight management programs are intimidating as they require excessive restrictions of food consumption patterns and are often compelled to warn against long-term usage. This is not true with the Food Lover's Diet. Using the Food Lover's Diet as your guide for weight loss, management and "braking" assures nutritional balance and flexibility for life.

Why not have a party and share the program with your friends? Jeanne Jones' book includes everything you'll need to plan your party. She establishes the flexibility for casual or formal entertaining while maintaining a healthy diet. Have no fears—Jeanne provides an eating pattern fit for a "king" which is also safe for those on modified fat, carbohydrate or salt diets.

I hope you enjoy *Food Lover's Diet* as much as I do and let it be your guide to a sound lifelong nutritional program.

BARBARA E. GUNNING, PH.D., R.D.
Professor, Family Studies and Consumer Science
San Diego State University
San Diego, California

Introduction

I love food. I love everything about it! I love to eat. I love to cook and I love to entertain; but I also love to look good, feel good and have lots of energy.

Have you ever stopped to realize that it is only when you are losing weight or successfully maintaining your desired weight you experience a positive feeling about yourself and everything and everyone else? Your psychological well-being is indeed hinged on the shape you are in—literally!

This is true whether you are only a few pounds overweight or truly obese. When you are gaining weight you have a low feeling of self-worth, as well as guilt for not being in control of your own body. How many times have you started to get dressed for a special occasion only to find that the outfit you planned to wear was too tight to button or zip? Even if you have something else you can wear, you don't have as much fun and feel ashamed of yourself.

Remember the time you didn't want to go on a trip you had been looking forward to because you hadn't lost the weight you promised yourself you would and so had practically nothing to wear? Or the time you made up a phony excuse when friends asked you to go to the beach because you were embarrassed about the way you looked in a bathing suit? This may have happened whether you were 10 pounds overweight and couldn't hold your stomach in, or 75 pounds over-weight and were afraid someone would ask you to play volleyball on the sand (you couldn't admit you're afraid it might kill you). We all go through this personal punishment and self-induced torment, wasting wonderful times, because we don't look the way we want to and can't perform the way we feel we should. How many precious days of happiness have you totally wasted wallowing in the self-deprecating despair of too much fat? You can't go skiing because the ski pants are too tight; or you can't play golf, tennis, etc., for similar reasons. How often have you said, "Next year I'm going to lose weight and everything is going to be different"? Then next year rolls around and nothing has changed, including your size? The saying "Today is the first day of the rest of your life" is more true than trite. Stop saying to yourself, "I wish I could lose weight" and start saying, "I *will.*" Stop saying, "I am going to go on a diet next week"—or "I'll get in shape before summer." This is living your life as though it were a dress rehearsal for the real performance. Unless you know something I don't, this is not a rehearsal for your life—this is the performance. You get up each day to give the final performance you will ever give for that day, so make it count—be the star you want to be. You are going to start enjoying looking good and feeling wonderful when you dress up to go out, whatever the occasion might be, because you will have learned how to stay thin *forever!*

When you feel fat and ugly, the accompanying self-pity will usually only make the problem worse—until you develop the resolve to lose the weight "once and for all"! Most people will then choose the current fad diet promising the greatest weight loss in the shortest period of time and they will stay on it until they can't stand the monotony and boredom of the diet or the restrictions it places on their social life. Often they develop a compulsive desire to eat things that aren't on the diet. They have not learned how to make the right decisions about food for themselves, so they go right back to old habits, regaining pounds and experiencing the mental anguish that goes with it. These diet ups and downs are called the "yo-yo syndrome" by behavioral psychologists. They occur because diets frequently restrict the very foods which give the greatest feeling of well-being—complex carbohydrates, things like potatoes, bread, cereal, waffles, pancakes and pasta. It is difficult to feel satisfied on celery sticks, lean meat, cottage cheese or even pineapple forever!

The Jeanne Jones Food Lover's Diet is truly a diet revolution. *Why?* Because it allows you to eat all of the "soul food" you want and restricts only the foods which contain fat and cholesterol. On this diet you will never feel hungry or deprived, and it is completely *safe!* You can stay on it *forever* if you like—and certainly until you reach your desired weight. Then, on the Lifetime Diet I have outlined, you can eat anything you want, applying only the rules of common sense and moderation. You will also learn the trick of *diet brakes* which will help you to stay trim and to eat without guilt for the rest of your life.

The excuses many people give for their diet habits are "I must eat out all the time," or "I travel constantly" or "I have to go to dinner parties almost every night and when I'm not at someone else's party I'm giving one myself." The late Bing Crosby, who traveled a great deal and was entertained royally in the process, was once asked how he stayed so slim. He answered that he ate everything he wanted but never all of it. You have the power—food doesn't. If food had the power to make you eat it, then everyone would be fat.

Most diet books tell you *what* to do but none of them tell you *why*. Also, most diet books take a negative, clinical approach. They have lists of things not allowed on the diet and still other lists of things that must be included in the diet. But nowhere can you find the reasons *why*. The *Food Lover's Diet* explains the reason behind everything you eat.

We are all much more willing to follow the rules if we understand them. The same principle is true of diet rules. Many diet books tell you not to eat butter or use salad dressings because they are "fattening" or because they are high in calories. Wouldn't you like to know why they are "fattening" or higher in calories than anything else? They also tell you not to drink alcoholic beverages when you are trying to lose weight, without explaining the reason behind it. I know one woman who assumed she would become an alcoholic if she drank while on a low-calorie diet, so whenever she wanted a drink she simply had more of everything else all day. No one had bothered to explain to her why alcohol was not allowed or why it was at least discouraged on a weight-loss diet.

There are many books on low-sodium cooking that tell you to cook without salt, but they do not tell you *how*. They do not explain the sodium content of foods nor do they tell you what sodium is, what salt is, how they are related or why controlling them is so important. They do not supply you with the secrets of salt-free cooking—tricks that keep you from missing salt. There are also many low-cholesterol diets available that never tell you what cholesterol is or what harm it can cause you—only to eat less of it.

Wouldn't you really like to know the answers to all of these questions? I know I did. Since cooking and entertaining are my favorite hobbies, I decided to fill this need by writing a medically sound diet book for people who love food as much as I do and who also share my enthusiasm for looking good, feeling good and having lots of energy to enjoy the other fun things in life.

In the *Food Lover's Diet,* I explain in detail the principles of good nutrition and weight loss. You will never again have to wonder why anything is important nutritionally for controlling your weight. This is really a nutrition education built into a diet, designed so that at the end of just two weeks you will know all about nutrition in general as well as particular types of diets. Plus, you are going to find that while you are losing weight on the Food Lover's Diet you will have more energy than you did before. You *won't* have that tired, listless feeling associated with so many other weight-loss diets. So get started today—learning *and* losing!

Remember how on other diets you always gained the weight back afterwards because you stopped doing what they told you to do without really understanding why? You did not know how to maintain a good diet program for yourself. After going on the Food Lover's Diet for only two weeks you are going to understand everything you need to know about designing your own diet program—in other words you will be able to eat and drink anything you want without gaining weight because you will have learned *how.*

Turn over the proverbial new leaf and start today on a lifetime diet that works—that will make you feel younger, happier, sexier and more important. Change your life with the Food Lover's Diet!

PART I

LEARN WHILE YOU LOSE

A NUTRITIONAL EDUCATION BUILT INTO A DIET

Food Categories and Groups

FOOD CATEGORIES

All foods are divided into three nutritional categories: carbohydrates, proteins and fats. Within each of these categories there are still further divisions:

CARBOHYDRATES
Simple carbohydrates
Complex carbohydrates (starches)
PROTEINS
Animal protein
Vegetable protein
FATS
Saturated fat
Polyunsaturated fat
Monounsaturated fat

CARBOHYDRATES

Carbohydrates are the major fuel source for the body. Carbohydrates provide the energy necessary for the body to function properly. In other words, the body is a carbohydrate-burning engine.

SIMPLE CARBOHYDRATES are the refined carbohydrates such as sugars—sucrose, fructose, maltose, dextrose, glucose and lactose—and syrups such as molasses, honey and corn syrup. These refined sugars are simple carbohydrates, containing no other nutritional value other than the calories available as carbohydrates, and should be eaten sparingly because they do not contribute to the total nutrition picture. Refined flours and highly processed cereals are also usually classified with the simple carbohydrates because most of their nutritional properties have been removed. When these highly refined products are "enriched," they do not get back any of their fiber. They are enriched with niacin, thiamin, riboflavin and iron.

The *sweetness* of fresh fruit and *some* vegetables is primarily due to the fructose content. Fructose is a naturally occurring sugar which is a simple carbohydrate. However, the *rest of the fruit or vegetable,* that part which is not made up of fructose and other sugars, is composed of complex carbohydrates, containing vitamins, minerals and fiber. Thus, simple carbohydrates eaten in the form of fresh fruits and sweet vegetables (for example, sweet corn and sweet peas) have nutritional benefits not found in refined carbohydrates. The sweetness of milk and other dairy products comes primarily from lactose, another simple carbohydrate. When some grains are sprouted, such as wheat berries, the result is a very sweet-tasting sprout. This is because the sprouting process converts wheat starch into the simple carbohydrate maltose. In fact, the sweetness of any food must come from one of the simple carbohydrate sugars, and the sweeter the food is, the higher its simple carbohydrate content; however, foods such as fruit, in which the simple carbohydrates are combined with other nutrients are more desirable for eating than refined sugar, which has no nutritional benefit other than the calories available for energy. This principle is called *nutrient density.* In other words, always try to eat foods that offer the most nutritional benefit for the calories consumed.

COMPLEX CARBOHYDRATES are of plant origin. Since fiber exists only in foods of plant origin and cholesterol exists only in foods of animal origin, complex carbohydrates are obviously important on a high-fiber, low-cholesterol diet. Complex carbohydrates are unrefined carbohydrates that also contain protein and sometimes fat. They are excellent sources of vitamins, minerals and fiber. Complex carbohydrates include all whole grains, unrefined flours and cereals, as well as those parts of fresh fruit and vegetables which do not contribute to the sweetness. Complex carbohydrate foods satisfy both the physiological and psychological desire for food. You never feel deprived. You have something of substance to eat that really "sticks to your ribs." Fruit satisfies the urge for something sweet, and it comes wrapped in beautiful containers full of vitamins, minerals and fiber instead of candy bar covering—and saves you hundreds of "empty calories." For these reasons complex carbohydrates are not limited on the Food Lover's Diet.

PROTEINS

Proteins are often described as the building blocks of the body. An adequate amount of protein is necessary for growth, maintenance and repair of body cells. Protein is available in one form or another in almost all foods. Most often, though, protein is associated with foods of animal origin. The problem is that many of these protein-rich foods are also high in fat and cholesterol, and therefore their amounts must be controlled in a healthful diet program. Animal protein is also a major source of protein in two of the three types of vegetarian diets. Vegan-vegetarians eat only foods of plant origin. However, lacto-vegetarians add dairy products to the vegetarian diet; and lacto-ovo-vegetarians add dairy products *and* eggs to the vegetarian diet.

When getting protein only from foods of vegetable origin, it is necessary to understand protein complementarity. This is a method of combining food groups within the vegetable-protein category to supplement missing amino acids. There are nine essential amino acids that cannot be produced by the body and must be obtained from food. If the proteins available are combined to make up for deficiencies in the essential amino acids, the body is able to use more of the protein. Combining proteins is not as important in diets containing adequate amounts of animal protein, which are already complete proteins containing all nine of these essential amino acids. More detailed information on complementing proteins in vegetarian diets and a chart showing the most effective combinations can be found in the chapter on the Vegetarian Diet.

Lacto-vegetarian diets rely heavily on dairy products as one of their main protein sources. All dairy products contain cholesterol. Most cheeses are high in fat and also high in sodium. Even low-fat dairy products are often high in cholesterol and sodium. Lacto-ovo-vegetarian diets have a special problem controlling cholesterol and fat intake because they usually rely heavily on eggs as well as dairy products for their protein. An average egg yolk contains about 250 milligrams of cholesterol and according to the American Heart Association no one should take in more than 300 milligrams of cholesterol per day.

Both lacto-vegetarians and lacto-ovo-vegetarians should rely more heavily on combining foods of vegetable origin that complement each other to provide the necessary amount of usable protein rather than relying so much on dairy products and eggs.

Animal proteins are limited on the Food Lover's Diet in order to control the intake of fat and cholesterol, with foods of vegetable origin providing the necessary additional amounts of protein and vitamins and minerals.

FAT

Although a certain amount of fat is necessary in your diet, it is not necessary to *add* fat to a well-balanced diet. There is enough fat available in the allowed amounts of other foods on the Food Lover's Diet to ensure an adequate percentage of fat in the diet. Fat is never added to any diet for nutritional reasons. Rather, it is used for flavor and texture in preparing salad dressings and marinades and for cooking and baking. It serves as a lubricant to prevent sticking when frying or sautéing and adds "richness" to sauces and flakiness to puff pastries and pie crusts.

Many people assume that fat improves the complexion. On the contrary, too much fat causes people to break out in unattractive blemishes, and acne patients are frequently put on low-fat diets. It is the moisture in the skin that keeps it resilient and youthful looking; drinking an adequate amount of water each day is essential for a beautiful complexion. Linoleic acid, the only essential fatty acid, is not an animal fat but a polyunsaturated fat, abundant in such complex carbohydrates as grains. Therefore, with a well-balanced diet containing adequate amounts of complex carbohydrate, there is no such thing as a fat deficiency; nor will you be wearing the fat in all the wrong places—on your stomach, under your arms or on your outer thighs! The excess fat you wear as padding on the outside is unattractive; you may even think it downright ugly. But the fat crowding your organs on the inside and clogging the inside of your blood vessels is truly dangerous to your health and your life.

For these reasons added fat is not permitted on the Food Lover's Basic Diet and it is limited on the Lifetime Diet.

SATURATED FATS include all fats of animal origin plus coconut and coconut and palm oils. It is believed by many cardiovascular physicians that the saturated fats tend to build up cholesterol in the blood vessels. For this reason I call them the "bad guys."

POLYUNSATURATED FATS are the "good guys." They include such oils as safflower, corn, cottonseed, sesame and sunflower. Many doctors feel that they tend to help rid the artery walls of newly deposited cholesterol and thereby enlarge the blood vessels and reduce the cholesterol problem to some extent. The highly polyunsaturated fats are all liquid at room temperature. Hydrogenating them will harden them, giving them texture. The harder they are, the less polyunsaturated they are. Tub margarines are therefore better than stick margarine. Pure corn oil margarine is considered by most dietitians to be the best choice in margarines and the most highly polyunsaturated. Many margarines are blended and contain coconut or palm oil, which are not polyunsaturated fats. Pure corn oil margarine also has a better flavor than the others when heated.

MONOUNSATURATED FATS are neither bad guys nor good guys. They stand on neutral ground because they neither help to build up cholesterol on artery walls nor do they help to rid the vessels of already deposited cholesterol. Monounsaturated fats include olives and olive oil, avocados and oils from nuts.

Since all fats have the same high calorie density, it only makes good common sense to select polyunsaturated fats for salad dressings and spreads and for cooking when given the choice. This is important to remember when you start the Lifetime Diet and begin adding some fats to your diet.

FOOD GROUPS

There are six basic food groups. All foods are divided into these groups according to the amount of carbohydrates, protein and fat that each contains.

FRUITS

VEGETABLES

STARCHES

PROTEINS

MILK (DAIRY)

FAT

FRUITS

Fruits contain primarily carbohydrates. They are important as a source of fiber, vitamins and minerals. Because they are sweet, they make wonderful desserts. They can also be added to other foods to enhance flavor and sweetness without adding refined sugar. Fruits are lower in sodium than any other food group.

VEGETABLES

Foods in the vegetable category contain carbohydrates and small amounts of protein. They are important sources of fiber, vitamins and minerals. They are truly the dieter's best friends—many vegetables are so low in calories when eaten raw that they are on your Free-Food List and can be eaten as snacks whenever you desire. Cooking vegetables condenses the carbohydrates, and therefore the same "free" vegetables, when cooked, cannot be eaten freely between meals; however, they may be eaten without restriction at meals.

Vegetables are also beautiful. They add both color and texture to your menus. Many people who think they do not like vegetables have always had them overcooked. Vegetables should be cooked crisp-tender—they are more brightly colored, have more taste, a better texture and retain more of their vitamins and minerals than their limp counterparts. If you object to the smell of some vegetables cooking, your problems are over. The minute you can smell a vegetable cooking, you know you have overcooked it! (See the Vegetable Steaming Chart in the recipe section.)

STARCHES

The starches contain more concentrated amounts of carbohydrate and protein than foods in the vegetable category. They include starchy vegetables such as potatoes, parsnips and yams, grains such as rice and cracked wheat, beans, lentils and legumes. Also included are breads, crackers, cereals and flours.

The unrefined starches—the complex carbohydrates—sometimes contain small amounts of fat along with carbohydrates and protein. They are excellent sources of vitamins and minerals and are very high in fiber. They are an excellent food source on a weight-loss diet because of their high fiber content. They are satisfying and keep you from feeling hungry between meals. They are satisfying psychologically as well because you won't be deprived of something you can "really eat."

The fiber content of vegetables may also have a calorie-sparing effect. Because indigestible fiber speeds up the transit time of all digestible foods through the gastrointestinal tract, some of the foods that would otherwise add calories to your body may not be completely absorbed.

PROTEINS

Protein foods contain protein and some fat. The proteins are divided into three groups, determined by the amount of fat they contain:

LOW-FAT PROTEIN:
7 grams of protein
3 grams of fat
MEDIUM-FAT PROTEIN:
7 grams of protein
5 grams of fat
HIGH-FAT PROTEIN:
7 grams of protein
7 grams of fat

Proteins are good sources of vitamins and minerals and essential for growth, maintenance and repair of body cells. The protein group includes cheese, eggs and egg substitutes, fish and seafood, poultry, meat and meat analogs (substitutes which are vegetable products) and vegetable proteins, such as tofu (soybean curd) and dried beans.

MILK

Milk contains nearly equal parts of carbohydrates and protein and is divided into three goups, determined by the amount of fat it contains:

NON-FAT MILK
LOW-FAT MILK
WHOLE MILK

Milk is a valuable source of calcium and riboflavin and contains many other vitamins and minerals. All milk is not alike in appearance; it comes in many different forms. You can buy liquid milk in cartons or in bottles or in cans, and powdered milk in pouches, boxes and cans.

Since only non-fat milk is allowed on the Food Lover's Basic Diet and it is also recommended on the Lifetime Diet, I will limit my discussion to this category. The term used, either non-fat or skim milk, varies from one state to another depending upon the dairy laws (also, low-fat milk varies from one percent to two percent, depending on the state). *Non-fat* is the more popular term and is used in most states. Non-fat canned milk is labeled "canned, skimmed evaporated milk" because it is evaporated or condensed. It has twice as many calories for the same volume as liquid, non-fat milk. In other words, one-half cup of canned, skimmed evaporated milk has 80 calories, as does one cup of liquid, non-fat milk. Non-fat canned milk is a wonderful product in a weight control program because it can be whipped to the consistency of whipped cream. (See the recipe for Whipped "Cream" in the recipe section.)

The powdered milk comes in two forms—instant and non-instant. The instant variety can be easily mixed into water with a spoon. The non-instant dry milk must be mixed in a blender. Dry, non-fat milk is a wonderful help for busy people. I always tell people it is just like having a cow in your own kitchen: Anytime you need milk, just measure out the dry milk and add water. One-third cup of dry, non-fat milk and eight ounces of water make one cup of non-fat milk. You may also want to use the dry milk with much less water for a thicker, more creamlike consistency for making sauces or for your coffee or tea. Milk may also be jelled for a thicker, creamier consistency when whipped. (See the recipe for Jelled Milk in the recipe section.) When cooking with non-fat milk it takes longer for sauces to thicken, so be patient—the time is well worth the difference in calories and fat content.

People who have a lactose intolerance are sensitive to milk and other dairy products and usually get a bloated feeling and flatulence whenever they drink milk. For them, LactAid may be added to the milk. This is a liquid which provides the lactase enzyme for digesting milk that some people do not produce themselves. It is available in health food stores and some drug stores. If it is not available in your area, write to the SugarLo Company, P. O. Box 1017, Atlantic City, New Jersey 08404. They promise to respond promptly and completely. Four to five drops of LactAid are used for a quart of milk, which must be refrigerated 24 hours before using. In some states LactAid is available in the dairy departments of food markets as ready-to-drink, treated milk. People with lactose intolerance can usually still eat sharp cheese. In the sharpening process, the lactose in the cheese is converted to lactic acid or lactate and therefore does not cause the same problems; unfortunately, sharp cheeses are usually high in both fat and sodium. For example, in one ounce of sharp cheddar cheese, three-quarters of the calories represent fat calories and only one-quarter proteins; and there are also 193 milligrams of sodium.

Milk is a wonderful appetite appeaser because it combines carbohydrates, which elevate the blood sugar, with protein, which stabilizes it. For this reason, on the Food Lover's Diet, you are told that you may use your milk allowance for midmorning and midafternoon pick-me-ups as desired; or, you may drink your milk about one-half hour before mealtime to take the edge off your appetite.

FAT

The fat group includes not only all oils, butter and margarines but also animal and vegetable foods that are so high in fat that they fit more appropriately in this group than any other. Dairy products such as cream cheese, sour cream and cream are examples of fats, as is bacon, which I list as a fat instead of a high-fat protein.

Vegetables like avocados, olives and all nuts and seeds are so much higher in fat than protein that they fall in the fat group. This makes them too high in calories to be used as a major protein source in a low-calorie vegetarian diet. They must be used sparingly, and only for flavor and texture, in any diet controlling calorie and fat intake. The vitamins and minerals in fats come packaged in very high-calorie "containers" and should be used sparingly as nutritional sources.

POLYUNSATURATED FATS, however, the "good guys" described earlier as helpful in regulating cholesterol build-up in the blood vessels, are also a source of the essential fatty acid, linoleic acid, without which the body cannot properly make fats. Two other polyunsaturated fatty acids, arachidomic and linolenic, are also important; the body, though, can manufacture them from linoleic acid.

SATURATED FATS serve no useful purpose and can be harmful to your health. Remember, they are the "bad guys" and can actually help cholesterol to form on the artery walls. They are not necessary in the diet at all, but they are present in all foods of animal origin to some extent. This is why added fats are not allowed on the Food Lover's Basic Diet and *all* animal protein is limited.

BALANCED AND UNBALANCED DIETS

A well-balanced diet is the single most important determinant of good health. A well-balanced diet is also crucial if a weight-loss diet program is to be safe. A diet that is well-balanced includes food from each food group every day. This ensures the body of getting all the vitamins and minerals essential to good nutrition. Without these nutrients, the body cannot function properly and does not have an adequate source of energy. A well-balanced diet also provides real food lovers with the variety of foods necessary for truly creative cuisine!

Many of the disease-prevention diet programs that are currently enjoying great popularity are indeed excellent diets; however, their promoters look at food solely as fuel for the body—"Eat it because it's good for you; never mind how it tastes or what it looks like." These rather spartan diets are for people whose social lives can easily adjust to a restrictive diet. The Food Lover's Diet is for people who, in order to be happy, want to adjust a sound diet to *their* life-style, rather than vice versa. The Food Lover's Diet is for people who really love food and enjoy the total experience of fine dining.

LOW-CARBOHYDRATE, HIGH-PROTEIN DIETS

Of all the popular "unbalanced" diets in recent years, the high-protein, low-carbohydrate diets have probably received the most publicity and have had the greatest following. In fact, some of these high-protein diets do not allow *any* carbohydrates at all.

The body is a carbohydrate-burning machine. Glucose is the body's main energy source. Glucose is the fuel for the brain and for muscles. When carbohydrates are not available, your body is forced to run on fat and protein—in other words it turns into a fat-burning machine. Fat burns inefficiently without carbohydrates and throws off a waste product called "ketones." This induces a state called "ketosis," a toxic condition that is potentially dangerous. It can cause nausea, vomiting, dizziness, low blood pressure and damage to the brain, and it certainly plays havoc with an otherwise sunny disposition.

If all of these reasons aren't enough to discourage real food lovers, ketosis also causes bad body odor and bad breath. One doctor, who acknowledges this in his high-protein, low-carbohydrate book, suggests using strong cologne for the body odor and chewing gum for the bad breath!

This type of diet can also cause an increase in the levels of uric acid in the blood which is very harmful to people with gout and arthritis. Moreover, these diets are high in cholesterol and saturated fats because of their reliance on meat, cheese and eggs, and raising the level of cholesterol in the blood speeds the development of arteriosclerosis.

When the body is relying only on proteins for energy, the protein is not available for its most valuable function, growth maintenance and repair of body cells, which can cause the body to lose calcium and thus bone as a result of demineralization. Also, when relying on proteins for energy, the nitrogen part of the protein molecule is left as waste material, forcing the kidneys to excrete large amounts of nitrogen waste. For a person with perfectly normal kidneys this is not a problem. But there are people with borderline kidney disease who don't know it until the kidneys are overtaxed; then it is too late. It can lead to uremic poisoning, damage to the brain and nervous system and even death in extreme cases.

Without fruit or vegetables, these carbohydrate-sparing diets can also cause scurvy from a deficiency of Vitamin C. In short, high-protein, low-carbohydrate diets are not recommended as a safe, sane way of losing weight.

LOW-PROTEIN DIETS

In direct contrast to the high-protein, low-carbohydrate diets are the many popular low-protein diets that contain extremely small amounts of protein and rely heavily on fruits, vegetables and grains. These diets are also unbalanced, and can cause deficiencies in essential minerals such as calcium, iron and zinc. When the protein intake is too low, the body is forced to break down its own muscle tissue for adequate protein, and you lose not only fat but also body mass and strength.

FAD DIETS

The fad diets include every crazy combination of foods you should eat exclusively or foods you should eliminate completely. Some low-protein diets, such as those that specify eating nothing but pineapple, papaya, grapes or watermelon, or only green vegetable soup, have all the problems described in diets too low in protein with the additional problem that they are deficient in essential vitamins and minerals.

LIQUID PROTEIN

The liquid-protein diet, which is sometimes referred to as the protein-sparing diet, was designed for truly obese people who need to lose 100 pounds or more. This diet regimen is almost a complete fast with just enough liquid protein to keep the body from using its own organs and muscles for its protein needs. This diet was also designed to be used under strict medical supervision—often in hospitals. The sudden popularity of this concept has led to many irreversible problems, such as abnormalities in heart rhythm, followed by death.

DIET GIMMICKS

I have often noted when lecturing on weight control that I honestly believe I could manufacture cardboard pills in a variety of colors and sell billions of them, giving the promise of overnight weight loss. Many of the "gimmicks" sold in abundance in this country today are not much better than my colorful cardboard pills. The major difference is that some of them are far more dangerous. Too many people get hooked on diuretics, or water pills, which can disrupt the potassium balance and cause heart rhythm abnormalities. Other people rely on laxatives, which can interfere with the absorption of many essential vitamins and minerals and also, as with water pills, cause a loss of potassium. Continued use of laxatives can also permanently harm bowel muscle function, leading to chronic constipation.

Amphetamines and other diet pills that supposedly reduce the feeling of hunger are also addictive drugs. You can become dependent on them because of their antidepressive effects. They are actually stimulants of the nervous system. Studies have shown that some of these drugs can also cause dangerous rises in blood pressure, even in normal, quite young people.

PSYCHOLOGICAL HAZARDS

There are the many physical dangers in unbalanced diets, as I have described. There are also psychological dangers. Many people who go on diets that are actually dangerous enough to shorten their expected lifetime gain all of the weight they lose back, plus a little more, as soon as they return to a more balanced way of eating. On an unbalanced diet, your body is not functioning properly and as soon as you go back to a more balanced approach to meal planning you are going to be putting on weight even more rapidly than you normally would consuming the same number of calories—which often causes depression. Also, you have learned nothing about how to maintain a good diet program because you didn't have the proper grounding. How can an unbalanced diet possibly teach you good nutritional habits? Many come right out and warn you that it's dangerous to stay on the diet for more than two weeks! The pounds you gain back because of this yo-yo syndrome usually turn up exactly where you don't want them—under your chin, in flab under the arms, in a bulging stomach, or in a sagging seat and the excess fat that looks like saddlebags on the top of your thighs—which is not at all attractive! Whoever said "Eat it today, wear it tomorrow" coined a good phrase.

The crazy thing about most people who want to lose weight is that they want to do it practically overnight. If you need to lose 20 pounds you must remember that you didn't put the 20 pounds on in one week and you aren't going to take the 20 pounds off in one week except through surgery, which is certainly not the recommended solution for fat thighs or a large athletic chest that has slipped and is now hanging over your belt.

VITAMINS AND MINERALS

On a well-balanced diet you are probably getting all of the essential vitamins and minerals needed for good health; however, it is a good insurance policy to take a covering vitamin-mineral supplement if you are concerned. (Iron, in particular, is important during growth and childbearing years.) With the exception of Vitamins A and D it is not considered harmful to take twice as many vitamins as you need, as they are water soluble. In fact, many Europeans claim Americans have the most expensive urine in the world because of all the vitamins we take. If you are in doubt about your own vitamin and mineral requirements, ask your doctor for advice.

Counting Calories

What is a calorie? A calorie is a unit of energy measurement. The potential energy provided by the various foods as they are metabolized by the body is measured in calories. One calorie is equal to the amount of heat or energy required to raise the temperature of one kilogram of water by one degree Centigrade.

Where do calories come from? Calories come from four sources—the three basic categories of food, plus alcohol.

All carbohydrates have 4 calories per gram.

All proteins have 4 calories per gram.

All fats have 9 calories per gram.

Alcohol has 7 calories per gram.

CALORIE DENSITY

The number of calories per gram of food indicates that food's *calorie density*. Understanding calorie density and the importance of getting calories from the best possible nutritional sources is the key to intelligent eating, weight maintenance and good nutrition in general. Understanding calorie density is also important for the real food lover in planning menus. When you want to come forth with all of your epicurean expertise and dazzle your guests with culinary creativity, you want to treat them as gourmets as well—not as gourmands.

The higher the calorie density, the smaller the portion size of food must be to control calorie intake. The lower the calorie density, the larger the portion size may be and have the same number of calories.

For example, simple carbohydrates, or the part of fruit and vegetables that makes them sweet, have a higher calorie density than complex carbohydrates, which are not sweet; therefore, the higher the ratio of simple carbohydrates available to complex carbohydrates in fruits, the higher the calories will be for any given portion. A sweet orange is going to have more calories than an orange of the same size that is *not as* sweet. This is also why a dried fruit, which is dehydrated and very high in simple carbohydrates, is so much higher in calories than the same size portion of the fruit when it is fresh. This rule also holds for vegetables. That is why one-quarter cup of peas has the same caloric value as *one-half* cup of carrots or beets or *one whole cup* of broccoli or spinach.

Just as you can learn to determine calorie density of a fruit or vegetable by tasting it, you can determine the calorie density of grains by the amount of fat they contain. In grains and grain products, the higher the fat content in relation to the complex carbohydrates, the higher the calories will be in any given portion. Wheat germ, for instance, has a higher fat content than does cracked wheat or bulgur. To receive the same number of calories, the portion size of wheat germ would have to be smaller than that of the other two grains. Calorie density in grain products is also determined by the relationship between volume and weight or texture. For example, if you are eating Grapenuts cereal, which has a very dense texture and is heavy for its volume, one-quarter cup would give you the same number of calories that you get in one whole cup of shredded wheat, which is not as densely textured and is lighter in weight.

PROTEIN FOODS

Protein foods, which are made up of both protein and fat, are divided into three categories according to calorie density. Calorie density indicates the percentage of fat compared to the protein in a food. (For additional nutritional information and exact portion sizes, see the Food Lists in the appendix.)

LOW-FAT PROTEIN
Each portion contains approximately:
7 grams of protein
3 grams of fat
55 calories per portion

MEDIUM-FAT PROTEIN
Each portion contains approximately:
7 grams of protein
5 grams of fat
75 calories

HIGH-FAT PROTEIN
Each portion contains approximately:
7 grams of protein
7 grams of fat
95 calories per portion

If you are a mathematical perfectionist and start multiplying the grams of protein by four and the fat by nine you will see that both the medium-fat category and the high-fat category are rounded off, and therefore the word "approximately" is used. The approximation is to make it easier for you to use the Food Lists when you start calculating your own calorie figures. You will find that all of the per-portion calories on the Food Lists end with either "5" or "0" for the same reason. The American Dietetic Association and the American Diabetes Association both approve of these figures for use by laymen—as well as by professionals.

Look over the protein lists at the back of this book. You may be amazed to find that many of the proteins you always thought were "diet foods" are in fact loaded with fat and high in sodium. For example, many people think of cheese as an ideal snack food because it is high in protein. One ounce of Monterey Jack cheese contains over twice as many calories in fat as in protein, and it also gives you 204 milligrams of sodium and 18 milligrams of cholesterol. Two-and-a-half Vienna sausages also offer you over twice as many calories in fat than in protein and contain 228 milligrams of sodium and 25 milligrams of cholesterol. Even in low-fat cheese, such as low-fat cottage cheese, almost 50 percent of the calories comes from fat, and in one-quarter cup there are 234 milligrams of sodium and 2.6 milligrams of cholesterol.

Studying the Food Lists I have provided, you will learn the calorie density comparisons very quickly. This knowledge will be of more help in determining appropriate portion sizes than anything else. You will quickly see that it is not just *what* you are eating, but *how much* of it that makes the calories add up.

PROTEIN FOODS VERSUS COMPLEX CARBOHYDRATES

When served a dinner plate containing a steak and a baked potato in a restaurant, almost every diet-conscious person eats all of the steak and very little if any of the baked potato. The irony of this approach to calorie counting is that the steak has probably four times the number of calories as the baked potato. This is because the steak, per ounce, contains approximately 14 grams of protein (56 calories) and 10 grams of fat (90 calories), or 56 calories in protein and 90 calories in fat, for a total of approximately 150 calories (in round numbers). Two ounces of steak is a piece about 3 x 2 x 1/4 inch thick—and when was the last time you or anyone else you know ate a steak that small? In most restaurants the average steak is about eight ounces, or approximately 600 calories. The average baked potato contains approximately 140 calories (30 grams of carbohydrate–120 calories–and four grams of protein–16 calories). Of course, this is assuming that it is served as it comes from the oven without butter, sour cream or chopped bacon. You know now that a rounded tablespoonful of butter contains 135 calories. So if you put a couple of tablespoons of butter and four tablespoons of sour cream (and another 90 calories) on your potato, it would bring it up to 500 calories; then, crumbling a couple of pieces of bacon on top of all that, it would equal the 600 calories in the steak.

Why is it that most people will always eat the protein on their plate before the complex carbohydrate? In my opinion it is because other diet books, written by people like Atkins, Stillman, Lin and the like, have made a world of dieters believe that the road to paradise is paved with protein. Indeed, I have found that most cardiovascular physicians would agree that eating a diet of bacon and eggs for breakfast every morning and fried chicken or a steak for lunch and dinner every day will indeed get you to paradise sooner than a diet that is higher in complex carbohydrates and lower in cholesterol and fat.

ALCOHOL

Alcohol provides only empty calories. There is no nutritional benefit gained by drinking alcoholic beverages; there is, on the other hand, a great deal of nutritional harm done by drinking too much alcohol. Not only does it contribute greatly to obesity because of its calorie content, but it takes very little alcohol to alter the judgment center in the brain, and you will end up eating foods you should not be eating, continue to drink more than you had intended and frequently feel terrible and guilty the next morning for having done so. I call this two-pronged problem the "double trouble" of alcohol.

Alcohol also lowers the blood sugar, making you feel hungry. The combination of feeling hungry and having less judgment about what you should eat is disastrous to a weight-loss program and plays havoc with weight maintenance on a lifetime diet. For these reasons alcohol is not permitted on the Food Lover's Basic Diet, and it is limited on the Lifetime Diet. It is not because you are apt to become alcoholic when taking in fewer calories but because alcohol contains seven calories per gram and provides no other nutritional benefits. Therefore it has zero *nutritional density* and a very high *calorie density,* neither of which you can afford when your nutritional intake must come from fewer calories. The story I told about the woman who honestly believed she would become an alcoholic if she drank wine on a low-calorie diet is not only true but also not as far-fetched as it might seem when you realize how many weight-loss diets tell you not to drink alcoholic beverages without bothering to explain why.

When drinking alcoholic beverages, dry wine is preferable to distilled alcohol because it is a "sipping" drink and usually is drunk more slowly. Three ounces of dry wine contain about 70 calories. Although one three-ounce glass of dry wine has about 70 calories, a wine glass this size is almost a thing of the past. Most bars and restaurants serve at least a five-ounce glass, which would be closer to 115 calories. The next time you think you'll just have that extra glass of wine that seems so insignificant, remember that it is just like picking up a roll and putting a rounded teaspoon of butter on it. No doubt you would think twice about buttering another roll if you were trying to lose weight, and the calories are the same—115. This particular comparison is a favorite of mine and it helps me refuse another glass of wine more than any other fact.

The calorie content of distilled spirits depends on the proof, and ranges from 67 calories for one ounce of 80 proof alcohol to 83 calories for one ounce of 100 proof alcohol (see the Alcohol Chart at the back of the book). When drinking spirits, don't order your drink "on the rocks." Have it mixed with bottled water, either sparkling or still, or soda. It is even a good idea to drink wine spritzers in which the wine is diluted with soda water. When drinking beer, choose light beers, which are lower in calories.

Alcohol may be used for cooking on the Food Lover's Diet because it evaporates in the cooking process.

FAT TRAPS

When lecturing, my favorite example of the insidious way fat sneaks up on you, adding calories to your diet from places you least suspect, is the relationship between non-fat milk, or skim milk, low-fat milk and whole milk. Imagine an eight-ounce glass (one cup) of non-fat milk containing 12 grams of carbohydrate and eight grams of protein and 80 calories sitting on a table. If you wanted to turn it into low-fat milk, you would add one pat (one rounded teaspoon) of butter. It would now have 125 calories because it would contain the same 12 grams of carbohydrate and eight grams of protein, but you have just added five grams of fat containing 45 calories. If you want to turn the low-fat milk into whole milk, you must add still another pat of butter, or another rounded teaspoonful. The same glass of milk sitting on the table contains 170 calories because it still has the 12 grams of carbohydrate and eight grams of protein, but it now has 10 grams of fat, or 90 calories available in fat. Do you realize that in one cup of whole milk you have three times as much fat as protein and twice as much fat as carbohydrate? This points up the reason why only non-fat milk is allowed on the Food Lover's Basic Diet and why it is recommended on the Lifetime Diet.

Another place fats overtake unsuspecting dieters who think they are righteously eating low-calorie foods is in sauces and salad dressings. It always amuses me to be with someone at lunch who orders a salad, telling me he is on a low-calorie diet, and then proceeds to pour five- or six-hundred calories worth of Roquefort dressing on the salad; or someone who invites me over for dinner and serves broiled fish because of a diet and then tops the fish with hollandaise; or the calorie-conscious "snacker" who orders popcorn at the movies because it is low in calories and puts one-quarter cup of melted butter (or more) on it. It takes three cups of popcorn to equal 70 calories, but just one-quarter cup of melted butter contains 540 calories. Conversely, one-quarter cup of popcorn contains about six calories.

It is easy to see why the Food Lover's Diet emphasizes the importance of complex carbohydrates and low-fat proteins. In the Food Lover's Basic Diet, added fat and alcohol are not allowed at all and they are limited on the Lifetime Diet.

With this information you can see that the old cliché, "Fat will make you fat faster than anything else," is completely true—and that fat can literally sneak up on you!

PORTION CONTROL

Portion control too is important to weight maintenance. You would not take your car to the gas station when it needs 10 gallons of gasoline and put 15 gallons in it. It would spill out of the gas tank, make a mess *and* cost you more money. But how often do you sit down at the table and shovel in twice as much fuel as your body needs or as your stomach can comfortably hold? The only difference is that it doesn't spill over— it bulges out in unwanted fat—*and* it also costs you money for fuel you don't need.

My favorite anecdote about portion size is one my friend and colleague, Dr. Morton H. Shaevitz, a clinical psychologist and Assistant Director of Bariatric Programs for the Scripps Clinic Medical Group, Inc., calls his anchovy story. A patient was leaving his office one day and asked him almost as an afterthought, "How many calories are there in anchovies?" He asked why he wanted to know and the man said, "Because I'm going out for pizza tonight and I wondered if I could have it with anchovies." Dr. Shaevitz replied, "If you are only having one piece of pizza it really doesn't matter how many calories there are in a few anchovies on the top—on the other hand, if you are going to eat the whole pizza it still doesn't matter how many calories there are in the anchovies on the top!"

CLEAN-PLATE SYNDROME

Get in the habit of always leaving a little bit of food on your plate. Too many people are card-carrying members of the Clean Plate Club. Most of them grew up being made to eat everything on their plate because of all the poor, starving children in Europe or Asia or wherever. Unfortunately, eating more than you should and getting fat from it doesn't help the poor starving children anywhere. When one of my sons was in nursery school, he was invited to a friend's home for dinner. After he came home he couldn't wait to tell me that his friend's mother told him he had to eat everything on his plate because of the poor starving children in Europe. Since he had never heard this before he couldn't figure out why his eating something he didn't want could possibly help anyone who was hungry in a place so far away. I told him that the next time he was at his friend's home for dinner and was told the same thing by his friend's mother to ask her, very politely, to wrap it up and send it to them. Well, of course you know what happened. He went back, and I'm sure even if he had loved his dinner he would not have eaten all of it just so he would have the opportunity to tell his friend's mother to wrap the leftover dinner up and send it off. And, of course, he prefaced it with "my mother said"! Fortunately, the friend's mother was a lovely lady with a good sense of humor who called me the next morning to say "thank you." She told me that her mother had always told her to eat because of all the children who went hungry, and so she figured that was the best way to get children to eat. It is this kind of misguided comment that has helped create a whole population of compulsive eaters in this country.

Restaurants usually serve portions appropriate for a man slightly over six-feet tall, weighing in excess of 200 pounds. If you are a lot shorter than that and shouldn't weigh over 125 pounds but still eat everything served to you in a restaurant on a regular basis, you probably won't grow any taller; however, you will undoubtedly approach 200 pounds! As the caption of one of my favorite Unger cartoons says: "Let me put it this way—for your weight you should be 37-feet tall."

A good motto in restaurants is "If you really want it, don't cut it out—cut it in half!" This way you won't feel deprived *or* guilty. (See the section on dining out for more tips on eating in restaurants.)

Also, don't become a garbage eater! Garbage is what is left on other people's plates. The next time you are clearing the table, put the garbage in the disposal where it belongs—not in you. It is not being wasteful to throw uneaten food away rather than eating it yourself. If you stop to think about it, it all ends up in the same sewage system anyway—only when it goes directly into the disposal or garbage can it doesn't make *you* fat.

CONSCIOUS EATING

After finishing a meal don't automatically eat dessert. Consciously decide if you are still hungry. So many people have what I call the "dessert habit." When they were children, dessert was always a reward. Remember—"If you eat everything on your plate then you can have dessert"? Looking back, it seems very funny that the part of the meal that is probably the worst for you from a nutritional standpoint was used as a reward. Nonetheless, such habits are hard to break and to many dessert still represents a reward at the end of the meal and it is a necessary ritual. How many times have you heard someone say "I just have to have a little something sweet at the end of a meal to feel satisfied"?

Start serving fresh fruit for dessert routinely, *and* then you can tell your children that they can have dessert first if they want it, and you won't be creating a lifetime association of rewards with foods that aren't good for them. Instead, give them non-edible rewards—like new clothing or tickets to the theatre or a ball game!

Choose what items on your plate you are going to eat before you start. You make conscious choices about everything else you do each day. You choose what you are going to wear, what movie you are going to see, what program you are going to watch on television. So start *eating* consciously. Make your choices before you start and then stop after you have eaten everything you have consciously chosen.

Saying "I can't help eating the things I know aren't good for me" is a cop-out. What you really mean is you won't. *Of course you can*— the question is whether you will or not. Some people wait to be saved with the kind of anticipation usually associated with religion, only they look for their salvation to come from the diet doctor, psychologist, friend or still another diet book. You are not a helpless victim. You are an educated adult and you can learn to make food choices just like you make all of the other choices in your life. You choose consciously what you want to wear each day—or maybe several different times during the day, when you choose to change into something more appropriate. You don't choose to wear formal clothing to play tennis or tennis clothing to a formal dinner dance. Then why should you choose to put lots of butter on your bread or cream and sugar in your coffee if you want to be thin? This too is an inappropriate choice.

In the consulting work I do for spas and fitness resorts, I have found that smaller-sized dinner plates are very helpful in controlling portions without making the guests feel they are being deprived. Also, eating with a three-tined fork rather than a four-tined fork slows you down. Eating slowly is important for several reasons. It takes at least 20 minutes for the blood sugar to rise sufficiently for your brain signals to let you know that you are no longer hungry; if you are eating rapidly, by the time the brain lets you know you have had enough, you may be much too full and uncomfortable. If you are trying to cut down on portions and gobble your food, everyone else at the table will still be eating and you won't have anything left on your plate. It will be very tempting to reach for another roll or order something else so that you will have something in front of you to eat too. Conscious eating, exactly as the term implies, means eating slowly enough to taste and enjoy each bite; it does *not* mean wolfing the food down so fast you can't remember a few hours later what you ate.

Behavioral psychologists have lots of other suggestions for slowing down your eating, such as putting your fork or other utensil down between bites, slowly sipping water or some non-caloric beverage between bites and practicing deep breathing before, during and after meals. All of these suggestions are potentially helpful; but the important thing is for you to eat slowly by whatever method works for you.

CALORIE REQUIREMENTS

Many people ask how many calories they burn each day. This depends entirely on your age, your size, your individual basal metabolism (your basic involuntary needs) and your activity level. It stands to reason that a man who is six-foot three and weighs 200 pounds and who exercises regularly is going to need three times as many calories to maintain his weight as a woman who is five-foot one, weighs 100 pounds and doesn't exercise at all.

To find out approximately how many calories you burn each day, multiply your weight by 12 if you are not very active. If you exercise regularly, multiply your weight by 14. Obviously, if you are someplace in between, 13 is a good compromise! To lose one pound per week, you must cut 3500 calories from your weekly total, which is equivalent to 500 calories per day. To lose two pounds per week, you must cut back another 3500, or 1000 calories per day.

To find your own calorie requirement once you have reached your desired weight, start slowly taking in more calories and at the same time weighing yourself weekly. If your weight starts to creep up, you know either you have to take in fewer calories or get more exercise, or maybe both. If you start to lose weight, you know that you should be taking in more calories. There is no way anyone can look at someone else and determine the exact number of calories necessary per day for weight maintenance; it depends on your age, your size, your individual basal metabolism and your activity level.

Once you are on the Lifetime Diet, it may help you to have a weekly outline so that you can plan ahead, eating more lightly or going back to the Basic Diet whenever you know there are parties coming up where you will want to sample the food without feeling guilty. Most food lovers also love parties!

Don't be fooled by the initial weight loss on many fad diets. It is not fat loss but fluid loss. By the same token, do not be discouraged if you start losing weight less rapidly during the second week. Weight loss has a natural downward curve. As you lose weight it takes less fuel to run a smaller body, and therefore you will lose weight more and more slowly at the same calorie level until you reach your goal weight. There will also be times when you do not seem to be losing weight at all. These periods are usually referred to as "plateaus" and the quickest way to get through them and start losing weight again is to take in fewer calories or get more exercise or both!

THE IMPORTANCE OF EXERCISE

Exercise burns up calories! Exercise not only improves the way you look by burning off calories, it also improves the way you feel. Ultimately a good fitness program will increase your self-respect and your self-confidence. You will stand taller, walk better and glow with the look of good health. You will even think more clearly. Putting it all together, regular exercise, combined with good nutrition, adds up to total fitness—a better mind, body and spirit.

The importance of regular exercise for weight maintenance has long been recognized. Regular exercise will help you to burn up more

CALORIES BURNED PER HOUR

(175-pound person)

LIGHT ACTIVITY OR NO ACTIVITY
Card playing: 100
Driving auto: 115
Eating: 100
Playing piano: 135
Reading: 100
Sleeping or lying still: 80
Sitting in class: 100
Standing still: 100
Studying: 90

MODERATE ACTIVITY
Bicycling (5.5 m.p.h.): 350
Bowling: 210
Busboy duties: 335
Carpentry, light: 255
Cleaning house: 280
Cooking dinner: 150
Crane operator: 255
Driving truck: 160–255
Fencing (moderate): 350
Gardening: 230
Getting dressed: 225
Golf (in a foursome;
walking, pulling clubs): 250
Horseback riding (trotting): 235
Making beds: 230
Pushing power lawn mower: 300

Roller skating: 350
Rowing (2.2 m.p.h.): 325
Secretarial work: 160
Swimming (20 yards/minute): 340
Table tennis: 275
Volleyball (moderate): 350
Waitress duties: 270
Walking (2 m.p.h.): 250

STRENUOUS ACTIVITY
Bicycling (13 m.p.h.): 760
Cross-country skiing
(10 m.p.h.): 1100
Dancing (strenuous): 400
Football (touch): 665
Jogging (5.5 m.p.h.) 750
Mountain climbing
(100 feet per hour): 690
Running (9 m.p.h.): 1150
Shoveling snow, heavy: 1170
Skating (strenuous): 700
Skiing (10 m.p.h. downhill): 650
Skull rowing (race at 20 strokes per
minute): 950
Squash, handball and racquetball: 700
Tennis (strenuous): 690
Trampolining: 875
Water skiing: 550

calories every day, and it also tends to depress the appetite. Exercise enables you to lose weight and inches faster and to maintain your weight and new proportions more easily.

Many people get discouraged when they start a good exercise program because the scale tells them they aren't losing weight as rapidly as they'd like. They are losing fat and building muscle. Remember—muscle tissue weighs more than fat and you may not be losing weight, but you are losing inches and growing smaller in size, which is, after all, what you're really trying to achieve—a smaller, better proportioned, firmer body.

Because of this very fact one of the major weight loss organizations in this country discourages its new members from exercising. Without the exercise, the weight loss that shows up on the scales is more dramatic and therefore is better insurance that the company will keep its members. At many spas and fitness resorts where exercise is stressed and where the change in body appearance in a very short period of time is unbelievable, people do not show a rapid weight loss.

CARDIOVASCULAR EXERCISE

Recently, the importance of regular cardiovascular exercise has been stressed as a way of preventing heart disease and promoting better health in general. Cardiovascular and aerobic exercises include all exercises which increase your heart rate. They include fast walking, jogging, running, swimming, bicycling, dancing and jumping rope. These activities strengthen the heart, enabling it to force the blood through the body slowly and steadily rather than in rapid, short pulsations that wear it out. The exercises all require exertion. Your heart beats faster and you begin to breathe more deeply. The blood vessels expand, carrying oxygen and blood to your working muscles. When your body takes in more than the ordinary amount of oxygen, you are burning calories more rapidly than normal. This continuous movement enables you to tone muscles and burn off fat at the same time. You should warm up slowly before any cardiovascular exercise or active sport, and you should always "walk it down"—bringing down your level of exertion slowly rather than coming to an abrupt halt.

The best way to measure your cardiovascular progress—and to be sure you don't overextend yourself—is by charting your heart rate or pulse. The lower your pulse, the more physically fit you are. Athletes, for example, have much lower pulses than less active people.

Your maximum heart rate (beats per minute) decreases with age, as is shown on the following Target Heart Rate Chart. It can be dangerous, though, to exceed 85 percent of your maximum rate, and it is preferable to limit yourself to 75 percent of the maximum for your age. This is called your target heart rate. Thus, by taking your pulse and charting your heart rate before, during and after strenuous exercise, you not only monitor the strengthening of your heart, but prevent yourself from straining it. As you become more fit, your resting heart rate should decrease and you should be able to exercise for longer periods before reaching your target rate.

Ideally, you should involve yourself in some form of cardiovascular or aerobic exercise for at least 30 minutes four times a week. This can be done in a variety of ways, ranging from purposely parking your car several blocks from where you are going each time you do errands, making a regular tennis date with friends or enrolling in a local gym or aerobic dance program. Keep a pair of running shoes in your car; then whenever you have extra time you can get out and walk or run. As an added benefit, you will be able to enjoy beautiful scenery when you happen upon it.

A wonderful advantage of regular aerobic exercise is that it not only burns up lots of calories during the time you are participating in it, but, because a greater supply of oxygen is going to your cells, your body will continue to work more efficiently *all* the time. You actually increase the number of calories you burn up per day on a regular basis. For this reason alone making aerobic exercise a part of your life should be very appealing! The "high" you feel after regular exercise and the "withdrawal" you feel when you miss exercise may be real and possibly similar to that experienced by drug addicts. But to my knowledge there's never been a "bad trip."

No one refutes the physiological importance of exercise. The regular walking, bicycling or aerobic dancing you do keeps you more aware of your body, more emotionally attuned to your physical well-being. It is a well-known fact among behavioral psychologists who work in the weight control field that people who purposely engage in regular physical activity have a much greater success in maintaining a desired weight after a weight-loss diet than more sedentary people.

TARGET HEART RATE

AGE	MAXIMUM HEART RATE (beats/minute)	TARGET HEART RATE (75% of the maximum in beats/minute)	TARGET HEART RATE RANGE (between 70–80% maximum in beats/minute)
20	200	150	140–170
25	195	146	137–166
30	190	142	133–162
35	180	139	130–157
40	180	135	126–153
45	175	131	123–149
50	170	127	119–145
55	165	124	116–140
60	160	120	112–136
65	155	116	109–132
70	150	112	105–128

PERSONAL HEART RATE CHART

1. Resting heart rate is taken just before going to sleep, without any stimulants or depressants—coffee, tea or alcohol, etc.—in your bloodstream. Feel your heart beat by holding your fingertips gently on the side of your neck or by holding them gently on the inside of your lower arm and count each beat as 1. Take your pulse for 10 seconds and multiply by 6.
2. Self-explanatory. Take your pulse for 10 seconds and multiply by 6.
3. Self-explanatory. Take your pulse for 10 seconds and multiply by 6.
4. Since the heart is a muscle, the cardiovascular time measurement refers to bringing the heart rate up to a target zone for the individual's heart to be exercised. This may be done by walking or participating in various sports.

5. Self-explanatory. Take your pulse for 10 seconds and multiply by 6.
6. Three to five minutes after your workout, take your pulse for 10 seconds and multiply by 6 to see what your heart rate has returned to. This recovery rate should improve as you continue your routine workouts.

	1	2	3	4	5	6
DATE	RESTING	BEFORE EXERCISE	AFTER WARMUP	CARDIO-VASCULAR	END OF WORKOUT	AFTER 3 MINUTES

IDEAL BODY WEIGHTS

Following are the ideal body weights, in pounds, for women and men 25 and over in normal indoor clothing. These weights are based on Metropolitan Life Insurance Company figures, and can be used as a rough guideline for your own ideal weight.

FOR WOMEN 25 AND OVER

HEIGHT		SMALL BUILD	MEDIUM BUILD	LARGE BUILD
4'	8"	89–90	93–104	101–116
4'	9"	91–98	95–107	103–119
4'	10"	93–101	98–110	106–122
4'	11"	96–104	101–113	109–125
5'	0"	99–107	104–116	112–128
5'	1"	102–110	107–119	115–131
5'	2"	105–113	110–123	118–135
5'	3"	108–116	113–127	122–139
5'	4"	111–120	117–132	126–143
5'	5"	115–124	121–136	130–147
5'	6"	119–128	125–140	134–151
5'	7"	123–132	129–144	138–155
5'	8"	127–137	133–148	142–160
5'	9"	131–141	137–152	146–165
5'	10"	135–145	141–156	150–170

FOR MEN 25 AND OVER

HEIGHT		SMALL BUILD	MEDIUM BUILD	LARGE BUILD
5'	1"	112–120	118–129	126–141
5'	2"	115–123	121–133	129–144
5'	3"	118–126	124–136	132–148
5'	4"	121–129	127–139	135–152
5'	5"	124–133	130–143	138–156
5'	6"	128–137	134–147	142–161
5'	7"	132–141	138–152	147–166
5'	8"	136–145	142–156	151–170
5'	9"	140–150	146–160	155–174
5'	10"	144–154	150–165	159–179
5'	11"	148–158	154–170	164–184
6'	0"	152–162	158–175	168–189
6'	1"	156–167	162–180	173–194
6'	2"	160–171	167–185	178–199
6'	3"	164–175	172–190	182–204

Diet Essentials

Most nutritional information about proper diet tells us a lot about restrictions, but we learn little about what makes a diet healthy other than that it must include all the necessary vitamins and minerals. Two essential components we should learn more about are fiber and water.

FIBER IN THE DIET—WHY IT'S FABULOUS!

We all hear a lot about the importance of fiber in the diet. In order to understand whether or not we are getting enough dietary fiber each day, it is important to know *what* fiber is, *where* it comes from and *why* it is important.

Dietary fiber is that fabulous indigestible part of plant food that is totally lacking in nutritional value, cannot be absorbed by the body and does not supply calories. In other words, it cannot make you fat. It does, however, add bulk to the diet because of its water-absorbing characteristics. In fact, the amount of dietary fiber available in a food is measured by its ability to hold moisture. As an English doctor I know says so elegantly, "It increases the transit of all other foods through the body." Our grandmothers often referred to dietary fiber as "roughage," but today many doctors prefer to call it "softage." When dietary fiber absorbs water, it swells, becoming soft and adding needed bulk for proper bowel function. Unprocessed bran, or "miller's bran," as it is often called, is currently the most popular high-fiber food supplement. However, it is by no means the only answer to increasing fiber in the diet. The best possible way to ensure an adequate amount of fiber is a diet high in complex carbohydrates (or unrefined foods), such as the Food Lover's Diet. Obviously, if dietary fiber works by absorbing moisture, drinking an adequate amount of water is important on a high-fiber diet. The Food Lover's Diet requires you to drink at least eight glasses of water a day!

Good sources of fiber are whole-grain flours, cereals and breads made from whole-grain ingredients. Seeds and nuts contain fiber, as do all fruits and vegetables. As the old adage says, "An apple a day keeps the doctor away." Remember that fiber is found only in foods of plant origin; so the next time someone asks you whether lamb or beef is higher is fiber, you'll know the answer is neither one—because they are not foods of plant origin.

To find out how much dietary fiber is available in foods of plant origin, check the Food Lists, which give the fiber content of practically every food. Not only is a high-fiber diet recommended for good general health and proper bowel function, research indicates it may prevent many serious diseases only recently associated with a lack of fiber in the diet. These diseases include ulcerative colitis, cancer of the colon, diverticulitis, diabetes and heart disease, to name a few.

An unrefined, high-fiber diet also offers natural protection from obesity. In his preface to my book, *The Fabulous Fiber Cookbook,* Dr. Kenneth Heaton of the University of Bristol Department of Medicine, Bristol Royal Infirmary in England, says there are three different ways fiber acts as a natural preventative to obesity. First, fiber must be chewed thoroughly before being swallowed and this slows down digestion. Whenever you slow down digestion, the brain is better able to respond to the rising blood sugar, letting you know you are no longer hungry; second, fiber is space-filling; and third, it promotes satiety, that satisfied feeling of having had enough to eat. That means you won't have enough room left for that last piece of gooey pastry— you're already full! Also, when you are on an unrefined, high-fiber diet, the foods you eat pass through your system more quickly than they would on a diet of low-fiber foods; thus, the body absorbs fewer calories, which serves as yet another aid in controlling weight.

There is an amusing aspect to all the recent attention being paid to the fabulous "new" high-fiber diets. Before 1870 and the invention of the roller mill, the same high-fiber, unrefined diet was the "old" diet consumed by practically everyone. Only royalty and the extremely wealthy were able to afford the small amounts of white flour produced because the process used for refining was so time consuming and costly. The majority of people ate coarse, dark breads which came to be known as "peasants' bread." To this day, this type of bread is still referred to as "peasants' bread" in many parts of the world.

The roller mill made the separation of the bran, germ and endosperm—the inner substance of grain—far more rapid and inexpensive so that an increasingly greater percentage of the population could emulate the upper classes and switch over to refined white breads. It took at least 50 years to discover that most of the important vitamins, minerals and fibers in grain were concentrated in the bran and germ which were either discarded or fed to animals.

In England during World War I and World War II, unrefined flour was used to stretch the supply of grain. A general improvement in health was noted during these periods, but for some reason it failed to arouse much interest or bring about any noticeable change in dietary education.

Another exciting part of this "new" high-fiber diet is how quickly it will become the way you eat by choice. You will actually prefer unrefined, natural foods, not only because in eating them you will feel better and find it easier to control your weight, but also because they are tastier, more interesting and add more variety to your diet than their refined counterparts.

THE IMPORTANCE OF WATER

Water will not make you rust! In fact, drinking an adequate amount of water will give you the glowing good looks associated with health and vitality. Whenever you are losing weight, your body uses stored-up fat for at least some of its energy, and it therefore throws off more toxins or impure body-waste products than at any other time. In order to wash these toxins or impurities out of your system continuously, it is necessary to drink lots of water. Drinking water helps your kidneys function more efficiently and also keeps your skin clear and more resilient and younger looking. When you are losing weight and *not* drinking enough water to keep the body's waste materials flushing through the body, the kidneys work harder, you are more susceptible to urinary tract infections and your skin breaks out.

In my discussion of fiber, I explained that dietary fiber is measured

by its ability to absorb moisture. It is this water-absorbing character-
istic that adds bulk to the diet; therefore, it is important to drink an
adequate amount of water when increasing the amount of dietary fiber
in the diet or the fiber can act as a plug in the system, absorbing all
available moisture and causing terrible stomach aches rather than
helping to speed the transit of food through your system. Water acts as
a natural diuretic, flushing impurities from your system, and it is
helpful in controlling water-retention problems. As strange as it may
sound, drinking water actually keeps you from retaining fluid. It's just
like priming a pump—the more water you drink, the faster it flows out.

Many people tell me they couldn't possibly drink eight glasses of
water a day. This is ridiculous. Drinking water, like any other good
habit, is just that—a habit. It can be acquired easily and become a part
of your natural life-style. To get started, I recommend buying a two-
quart plastic bottle and filling it with your favorite bottled water (or
tap water if you live in an area where it is not high in sodium) each
morning and making certain you have finished it by the end of the day.
Most people don't even take advantage of that first, perfect opportunity for a glass of water in the morning. When brushing your teeth
tomorrow morning, instead of simply rinsing your mouth out and
pouring out the rest of the water in your glass, fill the glass again and
drink it. Just think—that's one-eighth of the water you need to drink
for the whole day. You may even want to have a second glass, and then
you'll be one-quarter of the way there!

You can almost always tell by looking at a person whether he or
she drinks an adequate amount of water. People with clear, beautiful
skin are almost always heavy water drinkers.

The question I am most frequently asked about water consumption is "Can't I just drink more tea or coffee instead?" The answer is a
resounding *no!* The reason for drinking eight glasses of plain water
each day is to dilute toxic fluids and flush them out of your system. In
my discussion of caffeine, I stress the importance of reducing, or even
eliminating, all caffeinated beverages from your diet; they do *not* provide the same benefits that plain water does.

Many people prefer to drink a sparkling water. If you like sparkling water, drink a natural low-sodium sparkling water. Do not drink
artificially carbonated beverages such as soda water because they are
too high in sodium.

Diet Restrictions

Usually diet restrictions are considered to be only for the "sick," those who *must* restrict their intake of cholesterol, sodium, refined sugar, alcohol and caffeine. As a preventative measure, it makes good sense for *everyone* to apply the principle of moderation in these areas. None of these substances are required for good health—and all are *potentially* harmful.

CHOLESTEROL

Since we hear so much about cholesterol, I think it is important to know *what* it is, *where* it comes from and *why* we should control it.

Cholesterol is a waxy material present to some extent in all foods of animal origin. Egg yolk and animal fat of all types have a very high cholesterol content, as do the choice cuts of red meat that are marbled with fat, the skin of poultry, some shellfish and all organ meats. Also high in cholesterol are such animal products as whole milk, cream, butter and some cheeses. Cholesterol is found *only* in foods of animal origin; there is no cholesterol in foods of plant origin.

A limited amount of cholesterol is necessary for good health. When the body produces too much of it, though, cholesterol slowly builds up in the arteries, roughening, narrowing and reducing the size of the vessels through which blood must flow. This build-up along the artery walls is called arteriosclerosis. If enough cholesterol and other plaque material build up and actually interfere with the flow of blood in the coronary arteries, a heart attack or stroke results. A good analogy to what happens when this plaque material builds up is a garden hose that has become caked with mud. When you connect the hose to the water faucet and turn it on, the water cannot flow evenly through the hose. It comes out in irregular spurts and with great effort.

We *can* control the build-up of cholesterol. There are several ways. First and most obvious, cut down on the amount of foods containing cholesterol. The cholesterol content of these foods is indicated in the Food Lists (see appendix). Second, limit the intake of saturated fats, including all fats of animal origin plus coconut and coconut and palm oils. These fats can actually help build up cholesterol and other plaque materials. Avoid "non-dairy" milk and cream substitutes, such as imitation sour cream, imitation ice cream, cheese and whipped cream substitutes, unless the label specifically says "polyunsaturated fat." Most of them are made with coconut or palm oil, both highly saturated fats. If the label states "only vegetable oil," there is no guarantee that they do not contain coconut or palm oil.

The need to limit cholesterol in the diet was certainly reinforced in a recent news item stating that the Surgeon General of the Air Force had refused to accept surplus butter from the stockpiles of the Department of Agriculture because of concern over cholesterol. He decided instead to use all polyunsaturated margarines.

In most cases, high cholesterol counts can be lowered by proper diet; and everyone should be interested in preventing cholesterol build-up. Remember the old saying: "An ounce of prevention is worth a pound of cure." Even during pregnancy, good nutrition is an important factor in proper development of an unborn child. Babies should not be given diets high in saturated fats, cholesterol and refined carbohydrates. Start training small children in good eating habits. Children are not the ones who go to the supermarket and buy cookies, candies and other high-calorie-density, low-nutritive-density junk foods. Coronary build-up can start in childhood, so you should apply basically the same rules and diet principles to children that you apply to adults when controlling cholesterol, saturated fats, refined carbohydrates and sodium. You will indeed be teaching good lifelong eating habits. The nutritional principles followed in the Food Lover's Diet are ideal for the entire family.

TRIGLYCERIDES

Triglycerides are fats, also called lipids. We eat them in the form of fats and our livers manufacture them from refined sugars. When the triglyceride level is too high, the sticky triglyceride particles act like glue in the blood stream, causing the red corpuscles to stick together. These sticky little masses of red cells block the small capillaries so that the organs and tissues served by the capillaries do not get enough oxygen.

The most common cause of elevated triglyceride levels is excessive amounts of fats, refined sugars and alcohol in the diet. Also, such irregular eating habits as skipping breakfast and eating a large meal containing large amounts of fat and sugar later in the day can cause the triglyceride level to rise temporarily high enough to block the capillaries. Many people have experienced the feeling of being tired and lethargic after eating a large meal. This may be because the brain is temporarily not getting an adequate amount of oxygen due to the high triglyceride level. Alcohol will raise triglyceride levels as well, especially when accompanied by fatty foods. The same dietary and life-style habits that cause the short-term effects of elevated triglycerides also contribute to continuing dangerously high triglyceride levels.

The most commonly prescribed diet for lowering triglycerides is low in fat, refined sugars and alcohol. Also, regular exercise is important in controlling triglyceride levels. Some people misunderstand the link between carbohydrates and triglycerides. It is only the simple, or refined, carbohydrates—sugar, honey and syrup—that cause high triglyceride levels. The complex, unrefined carbohydrates such as vegetables and grains actually help control triglyceride levels. In other words, the Food Lover's Diet is perfect for people with high triglyceride levels.

SODIUM

Recently there has been much publicity about the importance of restricting sodium in the diet. I am delighted that it is finally receiving enough attention from the media to capture the interest of a major part of our population. In light of this new attention to low-sodium diets, I think we ought to know *what* sodium is, *where* it comes from and *why* it should be limited.

Sodium is a soft, waxy, silver-white metallic chemical element occurring in nature in combined form. When combined with chloride, it becomes ordinary table salt, the kind you put in salt shakers. According to the most recent Department of Agriculture figures, there are about 1938 milligrams of sodium (or almost two grams of sodium) in one *teaspoon* of salt. Sodium chloride is also found in foods of animal origin, such as fish, meat and poultry, eggs and dairy products. Sodium is found in varying amounts in fruits, vegetables and even in water. (The exact amounts of sodium present in serving portions of all foods can be found in the Food Lists.)

In fact, sodium exists in everything we eat or drink, with the exception of distilled water. I find it amusing when someone tells me, "I am on a sodium-free diet." What the person really means is "I am on a salt-free diet," which can also be described as a sodium-restricted diet. Sodium is sodium regardless of whether it comes from ordinary table salt, soy sauce, bleu cheese or celery sticks. It is ridiculous to be so hung up on the idea you are on a "salt-free" diet that you use soy sauce instead of salt whenever you cook. For one thing, you will end up giving everything you cook a slightly Oriental flavor—this is fine for Chow Mein or Eggs Foo Yung, but it is certainly less desirable in Beef Stroganoff.

If you are on an extremely low-sodium diet, you should not use either salt or soy sauce, or any other high-sodium product; however, if you are on a *controlled* sodium diet like the Food Lover's Diet for general good health, then you need only be concerned with the *total* number of milligrams of sodium you are consuming. By carefully calculating the milligrams of sodium present in foods, it is possible to enjoy occasionally foods usually considered taboo on sodium-restricted diets. This means that if you are particularly fond of celery, artichokes, Parmesan cheese, Worcestershire sauce, clams or even soy sauce and salt, you may use them sparingly, calculating the total number of milligrams of sodium in order not to exceed your doctor's prescribed limitation.

For example, you could put one-quarter teaspoon of salt in a cup of salad dressing, adding 484 milligrams of sodium, or put one ounce of bleu cheese in it, adding 510 milligrams of sodium—or sprinkle one-eighth teaspoon of salt on a baked potato for 242 milligrams of sodium, or mix two-thirds ounce of grated Romano cheese in for 247 milligrams of sodium.

In general, fruits have a low sodium content, while vegetables vary widely. Some vegetables which are very low in calories are high in sodium, so if you are counting calories as well as sodium, choose your vegetables with care. When available, fresh vegetables are always the best. When buying fresh frozen or canned vegetables, always check labels for added salt. Sodium can come from your tap water also. The sodium content of local water supplies varies greatly from one area to another. Check with your local water district, and if there are more than 30 milligrams of sodium per quart, it is advisable to use distilled water for both drinking and cooking. Home water softeners may be great for your laundry or for shampooing your hair, but they add a great deal of sodium to the water. This water should not be used for drinking or cooking. Many non-prescription laxatives, cold remedies, tranquilizers and headache medications have a high sodium content; check with your doctor before using them.

Sodium is an essential mineral, necessary in the right amounts for good health. One of the major functions of sodium in the body is working with chlorine to regulate the pH (a value used to express relative acidity and alkalinity) of the body fluids. In a properly functioning body, this is accomplished through a mechanism of the kidneys whereby chlorine is excreted when the body tends toward acidity, and sodium is excreted when the tendency is toward alkalinity. Sodium also regulates muscle contractions and nerve irritability.

Most people consume a great deal more sodium than is needed for proper body function and this excess is excreted by the kidneys. When the body is unable to get rid of the extra sodium because of diseases of the heart, circulatory system or kidneys, large amounts of unnecessary sodium accumulate. When sodium accumulates in the body, fluid accumulates along with it. The result is fluid retention, which causes edema, a swelling of the tissues. This is dangerous because it makes the heart work harder and causes the blood pressure to rise, a condition called hypertension. When hypertension is present, you must restrict the amount of sodium in your diet. Sodium's fluid-retaining characteristics have led many people to believe falsely that salt is fattening. Salt is *not* a food and does *not* contain calories, and it cannot make you fat; however, it *can* cause you to retain more fluid, making the weight recorded on your scale greater.

In the medical preface to my book, *The Secrets of Salt-Free Cooking,* Dr. Rene Bine, Jr., former vice-president of the American Heart Association, states, "A normal individual in a temperate climate, performing actively, needs less than 2000 milligrams of sodium per day (approximately one level teaspoon of salt). Needs increase somewhat in nursing mothers and obviously in cases where sweating is considerable. However, since sweat contains less than 1000 milligrams of sodium per liter (approximately one quart), in America more than 4000 milligrams would rarely be required except under unusual circumstances of location, occupation and hot humid climate. Yet the standard American diet contains around 10,000 milligrams of sodium per day and it is commonly much more due to the intake of salted snack foods!"

There are 1000 milligrams in one gram. Labels on low-sodium food products show the number of milligrams of sodium per 100 grams, which is about one-half cup. Serving sizes vary for each item, but the milligrams per serving and the serving size are also shown. Also, be aware that there are some diet foods found in the same section of the market that are for sugar-restricted diets only—read labels carefully for sodium content. The more you learn about the nutritional content of foods and about low-sodium cooking in general, the more fun you will have cooking, eating and entertaining even on the most restricted low-sodium diet, and the more you will be able to use your imagination in both developing new recipes and modifying old ones. The following chart may prove helpful in your experiments with decreasing salt in your recipes.

TABLE SALT	Mg. sodium
1 teaspoon	1938
3/4 teaspoon	1454
1/2 teaspoon	969
1/4 teaspoon	485
1/8 teaspoon	242

Exact amounts of sodium per serving portion are shown for almost every known food in the Food Lists. When in doubt, consult them. You will probably be amazed to see how high the sodium content is in many foods you always considered healthy snack foods, such as celery sticks and most cheeses. For instance, one cup of chopped celery contains 100 milligrams of sodium, while cauliflower contains only 12 milligrams; eggplant has two milligrams of sodium and 15 two-inch potato chips contain 300 milligrams. (Maybe that's why one of my friends always calls potato chips "salted fat.") Those salted French fries, usually with catsup poured all over them, you see people eating in fast-food restaurants, are loaded with sodium. Three tablespoons of catsup contain 564 milligrams of sodium. Four ounces of bleu cheese or Roquefort contain more sodium than a teaspoon of salt.

The major difficulty in developing truly delicious recipes for a sodium-restricted diet as opposed to other modified diets is that salt is a basic taste for which there is no real substitute. The taste buds on our tongue register four basic tastes. Starting at the tip of the tongue and working back, they are sweet, salt, sour and bitter. For this reason it is necessary to "fool" the taste buds into thinking that the flavor-heightening quality given by salt is present by overstimulating one of the other basic tastes. You are probably familiar with many recipes that list "salt to taste" as the final ingredient. That is because other than the four basic tastes, all of the "tastes" are actually *smells*. You will quickly discover that salt-free cooking adds a whole new dimension and importance to your sense of smell. If you don't believe this, hold your nose next time you eat one of your favorite foods and you will find you do not *taste* it. Do you remember the last time you had a bad cold and said you could not taste anything? Actually what you meant was that you could not *smell* anything, and therefore taste, as we usually describe it, was impossible.

We are not born with a desire for salt. Eating it is an acquired habit. However, from birth on we grow so accustomed to having our food "hyped" with salt, the great dietary whitewash, that we miss many subtle, delicate flavors completely. Low-sodium cooking is not only a new approach to seasoning, it is also a re-education of the palate.

The Food Lover's Diet relies heavily on lemon juice, vinegar, Tabasco and small amounts of pure crystalline fructose for flavor heightening, thereby reducing the amounts of salt used. To further enhance flavor, it is sometimes necessary to add up to three times as much of an herb or spice as you would normally use in a recipe. When using dried herbs and spices, it is essential to crush them, with a mortar and pestle, before adding them to the dish you are preparing. Crushing dried herbs and spices brings out much more of their flavor, or odor, if you will, stimulating the olfactory senses to perceive more "taste." To get an idea of the great variety of herbs and spices available to you as well as some suggested uses, see the Spice Chart I have included in the recipe section.

Salt-free salad dressings have a special advantage: They will not wilt your salads. It is the high sodium content in most salad dressings that draws the moisture out of the ingredients, causing the salad to become soggy. You can dress your salads with a salt-free dressing an hour or more before serving and still serve a crisp, crunchy salad.

Interestingly, the same property of salt that turns salads soggy can be put to advantage in other food preparation, without unhealthy side effects. For example, you can draw the bitterness from an eggplant by salting it and allowing it to stand for at least an hour. Then pour off the liquid the salt has drawn from the eggplant, rinsing thoroughly before cooking. This same method works well with cucumbers. When making flowers for garniture out of orange or lemon rinds, it is much easier to roll them without breaking the rind if you soak them first in heavily salted water for 24 hours—just don't eat the flowers afterwards!

FACTS ABOUT CAFFEINE

There are many good reasons to eliminate caffeine from your diet, or at least to reduce it as greatly as possible. Caffeine is a drug which stimulates the adrenal glands to produce more adrenalin. The adrenalin then acts as a stimulant, giving you a false high, or sense of having an energy spurt. In fact, caffeine actually *lowers* the blood sugar, giving you a *low* that is camouflaged by a false high for as long as the adrenalin keeps you stimulated. As soon as the effect of the adrenalin wears off, you have much less energy, since your blood sugar has been lowered, making you feel hungry. As you continue this cycle by again drinking more coffee for more stimulation as your blood sugar continues to drop, you get what is often called "coffee nerves"—you feel shaky, jumpy and your disposition probably is not as sunny as you would like it to be. (I have always believed that some genius figured this out years ago, and then came around to offices midmorning with a coffee truck to sell coffee to lower your blood sugar, making you hungry enough to buy one of his donuts as well. Then, by lunch, when the false high of the caffeine had worn off and the sugar high had dropped dramatically and you were starving, he came back and sold you some more coffee and some more junk food!)

Caffeine has other negative side effects; a well-known one is sleeplessness. In addition, there have been articles published recently that link caffeine to fibrous lumps or cysts in women's breasts. The results of tests now prove almost conclusively that by eliminating caffeine from the diets of these women these fibrous growths can also be totally eliminated.

Major sources of caffeine are coffee, tea, chocolate, many soft drinks and cola beverages. There is also caffeine in all decaffeinated beverages. When a decaffeinated coffee claims to be 97 percent caffeine free, the label neglects to mention that even real coffee is not 100 percent caffeine. Thus, decaffeinated coffee has less than six milligrams of caffeine per five-ounce cup, compared to regular coffee which has about 90 milligrams of caffeine per five-ounce cup. This means that drinking enough decaffeinated coffee has many of the effects of drinking regular coffee. A further problem with decaffeinated coffee is that some is still decaffeinated by a chemical process using a product similar to cleaning fluid. This process has been shown to cause cancer in laboratory animals. If you are going to drink decaffeinated beverages, make certain they have been decaffeinated by the Swiss, or water-washed, method.

All caffeine-free beverages are actually labeled "caffeine free" as opposed to "decaffeinated," a term you now know means only some part of the caffeine has been removed. Many caffeine-free herb teas are delicious. Start experimenting by buying several flavors so you can decide which you like best. Some of the more popular herb teas include chamomile, orange and cinnamon and spice blends. However, be cautious about unknown herb teas, as some may contain harmful drugs. Remember—water is the healthiest beverage in the world. Try hot water with a slice of lemon in it—you'll be amazed at how refreshing it can be.

If you have been a heavy coffee drinker for a long time and stop drinking coffee, you can expect to have headaches for four or five days afterwards. You are actually coming off a drug; however, I think in the long run four or five days of headaches are well worth the benefits of breaking the caffeine habit. Discomfort can be minimized by tapering off rather than quitting cold turkey.

REFINED SUGARS
AND OTHER SWEETENERS

Refined sugars should be limited on any good diet program. Fresh fruit is certainly the best dessert for all meals. I do not believe in the use of artificial sweeteners, as I see no reason for eating unnecessary chemicals, either from a medical or health standpoint. As far as taste goes, all chemical sweeteners available have a bad aftertaste when heated. Often when describing someone who is insipidly sweet, the comment is that the person is "saccharine sweet." This is certainly not a complimentary thing to say about a person, but I think it describes very well artificially sweetened foods which are insipidly sweet and leave a bitter aftertaste.

The most popular natural sweetners include sucrose (table sugar), fructose, syrups, honey and molasses. Of these, pure crystalline fructose is the sweetener of choice for several reasons. Fructose is the sweetest of all sugars—about one-and-a-half times sweeter than sucrose—and therefore you need to use less of it to attain the same level of sweetness. Fructose is sweeter cold than hot. The degree of its sweetness is also affected by the acid or alkaline content of the foods with which it is used. A good rule of thumb when using fructose is to use one-third less than you would use of ordinary table sugar; this also cuts calories. In addition, fructose heightens natural fruit flavors and makes fruit seem more ripe. Many people who always use salt on melon find that a pinch of fructose is an even greater flavor enhancer.

In fact, fructose is an excellent substitute for salt to heighten flavors. It may be used to season vegetables or added in small amounts to marinades, even when the desired effect is not sweetness. This is because, in the absence of salt, fructose will sharpen the taste of other ingredients. As I point out in the discussion of sodium, you must stimulate other taste buds in the absence of added salt. The combination of pure crystalline fructose and fresh lemon juice is the ideal flavor heightener on sodium-restricted diets.

But one of the most important advantages of pure crystalline fructose is that it does not cause the rapid rise and fall of blood sugar—and resulting hunger—caused by the high glucose content of sucrose and honey. This peak and valley syndrome is often called "sugar highs" and "sugar lows." The body converts all sugar into glucose to be used for energy. Those sugars already containing a high percentage of glucose enter the blood stream more quickly. (Sucrose is about 50 percent glucose and honey can be as high as 60 percent glucose.) This rise in blood sugar signals the pancreas to release insulin, which allows the sugar to move out of the blood stream and into the cells. You might say insulin acts as a key that opens the door to the cells. This causes a quick drop in blood sugar which then causes hunger. Fructose on the other hand contains almost no glucose and, because the body must convert it, the rise and fall of blood sugar is more gradual, as shown on the following chart.

COMPARISON OF INSULIN RESPONSES TO ORAL GLUCOSE, FRUCTOSE AND SUCROSE IN NORMAL SUBJECTS

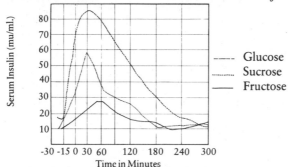

This chart is from an abstract presented at the annual meeting of the American Diabetes Association in Boston, Massachusetts, in June, 1978 by Nancy Bohannon, M.D., Assistant Clinical Professor of Medicine, University of California Medical School, San Francisco, California.

The comparisons shown on the chart are for pure crystalline fructose, which is almost 100 percent fructose. Pure crystalline fructose is available in almost all markets, either in the sugar section or the dietetic section; it is also available in most health food stores. If you prefer to use liquid fructose, you should know that it is not pure fructose, but is actually isomerized corn syrup and contains varying amounts of fructose along with other components, such as glucose, maltose, higher saccharides and water. Of the two most frequently used types of liquid fructose, Fructose 90, containing 90 percent fructose, is superior; Fructose 55 is only 55 percent fructose. Don't be misled by food and soft drink manufacturers who claim their products are fructose-sweetened. Most contain Fructose 55.

On diabetic diets, fructose must be counted as a nutritive sweetener. One tablespoonful equals one Fruit Exchange—40 calories and 10 grams of carbohydrate. For more information on the Diabetic Exchange Diet, see the chapter on Special Diets.

Remember—fructose is *not* a panacea. It certainly is not necessary in your diet, but it will satisfy your hunger for a longer period of time after eating it than other natural sweeteners. Also, it will make your food taste better than artificial sweeteners—which is important to real food lovers!

Many "sugar-free" diets use concentrated fruit juice quite freely to sweeten salad dressings, sauces and desserts. The sweet part of concentrated juice is also fructose. You are not saving very many calories or grams of simple carbohydrate because fructose contains approximately 40 calories and 10 grams of carbohydrate per table-spoon (three teaspoons); so, for example, concentrated apple juice contains 40 calories and 10 grams of carbohydrate in four teaspoons. You need to use only one-half to one-third as much pure crystalline fructose as you do apple-juice concentrate to achieve the same level of sweetness; you actually *add* calories by using juice. Also, if you use fruit juices routinely in your cooking, everything will have a slightly fruity flavor, which you may not want. In developing the recipes for this book, I tested every recipe containing fructose with apple-juice concentrate to satisfy my curiosity. In no case did I use it as an ingredi-ent in the final recipe because in no case did I find it as desirable a sweetener.

Many health-food faddists consider honey the ideal sweetener because it is "natural." They believe it is also an unrefined carbohy-drate. This is not true. Honey is a refined carbohydrate. It is refined by bees for bees; in fact, it is predigested food with a higher percentage of glucose than sucrose (ordinary table sugar).

One method of upping the perceived level of sweetness without adding *any* sweetener is to use vanilla extract and/or cinnamon. Skep-tical? Pour a cup of milk and add one teaspoon of vanilla extract and one-quarter teaspoon of cinnamon. Mix thoroughly and ask someone to tell you what you put in it. The answer is almost always "sugar." If you like sweet breakfast cereal, try adding a little vanilla extract to the milk you pour on it and sprinkle a little cinnamon over the top.

PART II

FOOD LOVER'S DIETS

Basic Weight-Loss Diet

You may stay on the Basic Weight-Loss Diet safely forever. During the first two weeks you may also want to use the Party Diet if you are entertaining guests or want to add still more variety to your diet. All of the recipes for both diets are in the recipe section. Or you may want to use the Vegetarian Diet I have included. You can mix and match parts of the Basic, Party and Vegetarian Weight-Loss Diets as you wish; from one meal to the next—or even parts of meals. For ideas, read Helpful Hints and Honest Cheating.

After the first two weeks, you may want to go to the Lifetime Diet program for maintenance or slower weight loss. On the Lifetime Diet program you are allowed to eat and drink anything; it offers you infinite variety and allows you to make your own selections within each food category in appropriate amounts. In fact, the Lifetime Diet may be the only diet you have ever been on which lets you literally eat and drink anything you want without guilt *or* regaining weight.

RULES FOR THE FIRST TWO WEEKS

● The only foods that are limited to exact amounts on the Weight-Loss Diets are animal proteins. Animal proteins are limited because they contain fat and cholesterol. You may eat less of them, *but do not eat more.*

● Limiting fruits to three portions per day is recommended to control the amount of simple carbohydrates you consume on your diet. In keeping to three portions of fruit per day, you will also increase the speed of your weight loss. To determine your portion sizes, turn to the Food Lists in the appendix. For breakfast, I have suggested a half grapefruit or an orange, the equivalent of one Fruit Portion.

- You must eat at least a little of everything on each menu. Do not eliminate any of the food categories or you will not have a well-balanced diet.
- Stop eating when you are no longer hungry. Never continue eating until you are full.
- Complex carbohydrates are not limited at meals and are, in fact, essential to the diets. Since complex carbohydrates are so satisfying and tend to be more filling than other foods, if you only eat until you are no longer hungry, these starchy foods will not impede weight loss. The important thing is not to stuff yourself!
- Eat slowly. You are less likely to overeat (see the discussion of portion control).
- Do not add any fats (butter, margarine, oil, commercial salad dressing, etc.) to your Weight-Loss Diet.
- Use only very lean meat and remove all visible fat before eating. Remove skin and fat from turkey and chicken before eating. Prepare all meat, poultry and fish without added fat, such as butter or margarine. Broil, bake, poach, steam or sauté (in the sense of cooking in a skillet) in non-stick cookware.
- Prepare all vegetables without butter, margarine or oil. Steam vegetables (see Steaming Chart), cook them in a microwave oven or sauté them in a skillet or a wok with a little fat-free stock. Lemon juice, fat-free stock, herbs and spices may be used for seasoning. Other fat-free, low-calorie condiments such as soy sauce, Worcestershire sauce, Liquid Smoke and Bakon Seasoning may be used in moderation, although some are high in sodium.
- Prepare all salads without oil, mayonnaise or commercial dressings. Use only vinegar, lemon juice or one of the Jones Salad Dressings I have included.
- Do not drink any alcoholic beverages. Try the Counterfeit Cocktail in the recipe section.
- Drink eight glasses of water a day.
- Herb teas without caffeine are better than regular coffee or tea (see the section on caffeine.)
- Between meals you may eat as much of the foods on the following Free-Food List as you wish.

● You may want to save your milk allowance for midmorning and midafternoon pick-me-ups instead of drinking it with meals or using it for sauces and dips. You may also substitute 1/2 cup non-fat yogurt for your non-fat milk; or 1/4 cup low-fat cottage cheese, hoop cheese or skimmed ricotta cheese. This affords you a great deal of variety in preparing spreads for bread and rolls, sauces and dips for vegetables, as well as sauces for fish, poultry and meat (see the menus in the Party Diet section).

FREE FOODS (WHEN EATEN RAW)

Alfalfa sprouts	Collards	Parsley
Asparagus	Cilantro	Peppers, green and red
Bean sprouts	Cucumber	Poke
Broccoli	*Dandelion greens	Radishes
Brussels sprouts	Endive	Rhubarb
Cabbage	Escarole	Romaine lettuce
Cauliflower	Green onion tops	Spinach
*Celery	Kale	Summer squash
*Chard	Lettuce	Watercress
Chicory	Mint	Zucchini squash
Chilies	Mushrooms	
Chives	Mustard, fresh	*High sodium content

HELPFUL HINTS AND HONEST CHEATING

You may mix and match recipes and ideas between the Food Lover's Basic Diet and the Party Diet as you wish. The following are some examples. You may wish to make Breakfast Cheese to have on your toast at breakfast every day or on your baked potato. You may substitute your milk allowance for cottage cheese and have it as a dip for your raw vegetables at lunch every day. You may make the Dill Sauce listed for the fish on Monday and use it as a dip for your relish tray later in the week in place of your milk at a meal.

You may always use the Marinara Sauce recipe as a sauce for pasta, vegetables and baked potatoes. It is also a good sauce for fish, poultry and meat. Instead of serving your pasta hot, you may wish to marinate it, along with assorted cooked vegetables, in the Jones Tarragon or Italian Dressing, and serve it cold as a salad. Since you can have cottage cheese for lunch on any day, you might try pasta salad tossed with cottage cheese. It's wonderful—honest! Chicken, turkey or fish can be added to the Pasta Primavera in place of the cottage cheese as another variation. You may wish to substitute the vegetarian entrées on the Vegetarian Diet for those on the Basic Diet or for the Party Diet. You may want to make Mustard Dip and have it on a baked potato and skip your milk for that meal. Chow Mein vegetables and noodles, without the seafood, can be used as a vegetable for any meal.

I have listed a specific vegetable for every meal, again to show you the infinite variety of fresh vegetables available and hopefully to get you to try new vegetables you may not have eaten before; however, if a vegetable listed is not in season and therefore not available fresh, or if a vegetable listed is something you particularly do not like, then substitute an available vegetable that you do like.

All vegetables may be sautéed in stock with onions for more flavor. Use your imagination. Adding grated fresh ginger, garlic cloves or any other herb or spice you like will give a great deal of flavor to your vegetables when you sauté or cook them in a wok in fat-free stock. Experiment with seasonings. For ideas, look at the Herb and Spice Chart.

The importance of complex carbohydrates is evident in this diet program, and you are free to substitute any of the acceptable complex carbohydrates for another. I mention a specific type of bread, starchy vegetable, grain, cereal or pasta for each meal to give you an idea of the nearly infinite variety available. On the diet program, I specify "whole-grain bread" as a substitute because it is almost always available; however, if you are in a restaurant where they do not have brown rice, bulgur or whole-grain bread, you could probably order a baked potato, which would be a perfectly acceptable substitute for the specified complex carbohydrate. You do not have to confine your cereal to breakfast either. If you would rather have a bowl of cereal with non-fat milk and fruit on it for lunch, there is no reason why you can't.

A relish tray, not limited to the vegetables on the Free-Food List, is specified for lunch every day because it can so easily be put in a bag for a portable lunch. Also, at dinner every night a tossed salad is listed, but a fresh relish tray with a Mock Sour Cream Dip may be substituted;

or you can have a salad for lunch if you prefer. Remember that your dip must always be counted toward your milk allowance for that day, unless you have it instead of cottage cheese at lunch.

I find that many people who work or go to school must carry lunch with them at least five days a week. Remember, you can substitute one-quarter cup of cottage cheese for your milk whenever you wish. This may be helpful in making your lunches easier to carry with you. You may want to use your milk allowance to make the Mock Sour Cream Dips to use as sandwich spread and combine them with the other ingredients that are allowed for lunch each day. For example, on Tuesday you may wish to spread the dip on your whole-grain bread and add sliced tomatoes, lettuce and tuna for a super tuna sandwich. You can also make wonderful sandwiches with either fruit and cottage cheese or vegetables and cottage cheese. Try a cottage cheese and banana sandwich on whole-wheat bread. Sprinkle a little cinnamon on the sliced banana or mix it with the cottage cheese. Also, you might try a cottage cheese and sliced tomato sandwich with lettuce. I like cottage cheese with chopped tomatoes and sliced mushrooms and alfalfa sprouts in a whole-wheat pita pocket. Try sprinkling a little Jones Dressing on the pita sandwich or a little Mustard Dip. It's delicious. Try a sandwich made with Curry Dip. Since it is a cottage cheese-based dip, you can use the cottage cheese allowance and it makes a delicious sandwich. A whole-wheat bagel with Breakfast Cheese and sliced apple is a real gourmet treat. In other words, when combining the simple, straightforward foods listed on the Food Lover's Basic Diet, use your imagination for ways to give you variety in taste, texture and appearance. Variety is indeed the spice of life, and imagination is the key to variety in your diet.

NON-STICK COOKWARE

For much of your low-fat cooking you will need non-stick pans. Generally I prefer "cured" heavy iron skillets over Teflon; they are better for browning and I don't have to worry about scratching them. To cure an iron skillet, take your new iron skillet (or your grandmother's old one) and put several tablespoons of oil in it. Place the skillet over moderate heat and when it starts to get hot, tilt it from side to side until the oil coats the entire inner surface of the skillet. Continue heating the skillet until the oil starts to smoke. Then turn the heat off and cool the skillet. When it's cool enough to handle, wipe all the oil out with paper towels. Repeat this process three or four times and you have a "cured" pan ready to use.

Never wash a "cured" pan with water. When you are through with it, each time wipe it out with oil. If food sticks to the bottom, rub it off with salt. If it is so bad that you have to wash it with water, or if you use the skillet to cook liquids, all is not lost. Do not throw the pan away because it looks rusty, *just cure it again!*

THINK STOCK—THINK THIN!

Whenever your first thought is to add butter, either for serving or cooking, think stock instead. There is nothing more delicious on a baked potato than a few tablespoons of beef or chicken stock. When using a recipe specifying butter or oil for sautéing vegetables or meats, simply substitute stock in the recipe. The same mixtures of herbs and spices and other condiments that can be added to butter can also be combined with stock for a lighter, even more delicious result, and certainly with a lower calorie, healthier result. Try the Herbed Vegetable Medley recipe.

It is so easy to make your own stocks once you get in the habit of doing it that I have provided recipes for both chicken and beef stock, as well as a vegetable stock (see Stocks, Sauces and Toppings). You can either buy the chicken pieces and beef bones necessary for the stock or talk your butcher into giving them to you; or you can do as French housewives do, storing up your bones in bags in the freezer and, once you have enough of them, making a pot of stock. Then freeze the stock in the container sizes you most frequently need or in ice-cube trays, using it as required for cooking (two ice cubes equal one-quarter cup of stock). When you make your own stock, you know it's totally fat free, and you can also control the amount of salt. Finally, you will find your own stocks are more flavorful and *much* less expensive.

However, if you are simply not interested in making stock, you can buy stock base, bouillon cubes or canned broth. The problem with most stock bases and bouillon cubes is that they are extremely high in sodium. When buying the canned broth, keep the cans in your refrigerator where the fat will rise to the top and can be easily removed. As you open each can, carefully skim off all fat.

WEIGHT LOSS RECORD

DAY	WEIGHT	
	WEEK 1	WEEK 2
First		
Second		
Third		
Fourth		
Fifth		
Sixth		
Seventh		

SUMMARY

Starting weight   ———

Ending weight   ———

Two week loss   ———

EATING HABITS

Practice conscious eating. Think about your food while you're eating it. Eat slowly, savoring each bite and thinking about the taste. You will find you enjoy your food much more and are truly satisfied with smaller amounts. As I'm sure you have heard many times, there is a real reason why eating slowly is a great aid in weight reduction. It takes time for the blood sugar to rise enough for the brain to register it and send the message to the digestive system that you are no longer hungry. You may have had an experience where you ate large quantities of food very rapidly and then felt too full for a long time afterward. You were literally taking in more fuel than your body needed and were uncomfortable because of it.

Conscious eating is the exact opposite of unconscious eating. How often have you eaten a whole can of nuts or bag of corn chips without even being able to remember what they tasted like while you were eating them? You have probably consumed hundreds and maybe even thousands of calories without enjoying them.

Never eat standing up when you can avoid it. Take the time to sit down and think about what you are going to eat and how much you are going to enjoy it before you start. Take a few deep breaths, drink some water and really plan to enjoy the meal you are about to eat.

Remember: The urge to binge never lasts longer than 20 minutes; so when you feel the urge to eat something you shouldn't, get away from it. This may mean getting out of the house or office and going for a walk, calling a friend or taking in a show—*anything* but eating!

BREAKFAST

BREAKFAST EVERY DAY

1/2 grapefruit or 1 orange
Whole-grain bread or whole-grain cereal
1/2 cup non-fat milk or plain non-fat yogurt;
or 1/4 cup low-fat cottage cheese,
hoop cheese or partially skimmed ricotta cheese
Coffee or tea

Since the basic ingredients for breakfast are the same every morning, these Breakfast Helpers may be useful in adding variety to your morning meals on the Food Lover's Diet:

If you do not have a lot of time in the morning, you may wish to make a breakfast shake. I like to make an Orange Smoothie, combining the orange, 1/2 cup of non-fat milk and 1/2 teaspoon of vanilla extract in a blender container and blending until smooth. If you wish a thicker drink, add some crushed ice to the blender container with the other ingredients. You can add some whole-grain breakfast cereal to the blender container and have your entire breakfast in a glass; or you may want to have a slice of whole-grain toast or roll with it.

If you are having cereal, you will want to pour your milk over it. However, if you are having bread or a roll, you may wish to spread cottage cheese on it. One of my favorite breakfasts is whole-wheat toast spread with cottage cheese, especially when I travel, because these ingredients are almost always available. When I am home, I sometimes spread a teaspoon or two of Jones Apple Butter on it. The recipe for Apple Butter is in the section on Desserts and Fruit. (For maximum weight loss, use the Apple Butter sparingly.) Or, instead of cottage cheese, ricotta cheese or hoop cheese, you may wish to use the Breakfast Cheese recipe (in the recipe section) as a spread. You may want to have sliced banana, strawberries or peach on your cereal in the morning rather than an orange or half grapefruit. If you do, simply substitute the grapefruit or orange for your fruit at lunch or dinner. Broiled grapefruit served warm is both an excellent appetizer and an unusual dessert. The reason I specify grapefruit or orange at breakfast each day is that citrus fruit provides an excellent source of Vitamin C, needed on a daily basis, and it is always available in restaurants in the morning, though it may not be available at other times during the day.

MONDAY

MONDAY LUNCH

Raw vegetable relish tray or bag of vegetables
1/2 cup low-fat cottage cheese,
hoop cheese or partially skimmed ricotta cheese
Fresh fruit
Whole-grain bread or whole-grain pasta
Coffee or tea

Monday's lunch may be used for lunch every day. You can easily carry it with you, and it is almost always available in restaurants if you are eating out. There is tremendous variety built into these few simple ingredients. At home, you may want to have a big tossed green salad with loads of lettuce and all the vegetables you might normally put on the relish tray, chopping them up and adding them to a salad. (For your relish tray, you may use any raw vegetable, not limiting yourself to those vegetables on the Free-Food List. For example, you may want to include carrot sticks, jicama and cherry tomatoes, which are not on the Free-Food List.) Then you could make one of the Mock Sour Cream

Dips out of the 1/2 cup of cottage cheese available for lunch and use it as a salad dressing; or you might spread the cottage cheese on whole-grain toast or a whole-wheat English muffin to have with your salad; or you might combine your fruit and cottage cheese for a fruit and cottage cheese salad, using one of the Jones Salad Dressings on top. You could also use the partially skimmed ricotta cheese and make open-faced sandwiches with whole-grain toast and sliced apples sprinkled with cinnamon.

A favorite luncheon dish of mine is the cold pasta salad I described in Helpful Hints. I marinate all my leftover cooked vegetables in the refrigerator in either Jones Tarragon or Italian Dressing and then toss them along with the cottage cheese and the pasta. On a really cold day, you might cook all of the vegetables from your relish tray in defatted chicken stock for a delicious vegetable soup, and serve it with toasted pumpernickel bagels spread with the Breakfast Cheese and a touch of Jones Apple Butter. Recipes for both are in the recipe section.

For each day I have a suggestion for a portable picnic or brown bag lunch which can be eaten without utensils. In this case, I like to make the cottage cheese into one of the Mock Sour Cream Dips and spread it on whole-grain bread with lettuce and vegetables, or combine ricotta cheese with apples or bananas for a fruit and cheese sandwich, and carry a bag of raw vegetables to have with it. If you are making vegetable sandwiches, you might want to substitute your fruit for the bananas on the Monday Dinner menu in order to take a banana in your lunch. Bananas are wonderful for brown bag lunches because they come in their own wrappers—all you do is peel and eat. Apples and grapes are also good for brown bag lunches; some other fruits tend to be a bit messy for practical portability.

MONDAY DINNER

Tossed salad (as much of any of the fresh greens
or vegetables on your Free-Food List as desired)
with lemon juice, vinegar or a Jones Dressing
4 ounces broiled or poached fish or seafood
Brown or wild rice or whole-grain bread
Banana or available fresh fruit
1/2 cup non-fat milk or plain non-fat yogurt
Coffee or tea

If you want to prepare dinner in advance, you might make a rice and fish casserole. Use the recipe for Brown Rice Pilaf and combine it with diced cooked fish and vegetables. This is also a good way to use leftover fish and vegetables. For dessert, broil a banana and sprinkle a little cinnamon on it and serve it with yogurt. You may want to make a seafood salad instead. Try tossing cooked shrimp through the salad and use your milk allowance for 1/4 cup of the Curry Dip as a dressing for the salad. Also, cold rice is wonderful in salads. If you are using the Curry Dressing, try blending it with the banana. You will be delightfully surprised with this marvelous banana-curry dressing.

TUESDAY

TUESDAY LUNCH

Raw vegetable relish tray or bag of vegetables
1/2 cup water-packed tuna
Tomato
Whole-grain bread
Strawberries or available fresh fruit
1/2 cup non-fat milk or plain non-fat yogurt
Coffee or tea

In Helpful Hints, I suggest a super tuna sandwich for this lunch: Spread the bread with Dill Dip and then add the tuna, lettuce and tomatoes. You could also have a large tuna salad with Jones Pineapple-Ginger Dressing and Jelled Milk or Whipped "Cream" on your strawberries. If you are particularly fond of cereal and had toast for breakfast, you may want to use your bread allowance for 1/4 cup of Grapenuts with strawberries and milk for dessert.

TUESDAY DINNER

Tossed salad (as much of any of the fresh greens
or vegetables on your Free-Food List as desired)
with lemon juice, vinegar or a Jones Dressing
1 baked or poached chicken breast without skin or
3 ounces white turkey meat without skin
Steamed broccoli or other fresh green vegetable
Corn on the cob, brown rice or bulgur
Melon or available fresh fruit
Coffee or tea

Try using the Chicken in Envelopes recipe and pour the juice from the envelope on the corn on the cob as well as the broccoli. It's delicious. Or you might enjoy a chicken and broccoli casserole. Combine chopped chicken and chopped broccoli with the cooked bulgur and chicken stock and a little crushed dried tarragon. This is a wonderful way to use leftovers and can be made ahead of time. Another possibility is the recipe for Lemon Bulgur, with the addition of the chicken and broccoli. Try spreading Mustard Dip on your corn on the cob. You will love it! Either cut your melon into bite-sized pieces or make it into melon balls and sprinkle lightly with ground aniseed for a really unusual taste treat. If you don't like anise, use a little ground cinnamon.

WEDNESDAY

WEDNESDAY LUNCH

Raw vegetable relish tray or bag of vegetables
Tossed lettuce and tomato salad
with lemon juice, vinegar or a Jones Dressing
1 dozen *small* cooked shrimp or 1/2 cup water-packed tuna
Papaya or available fresh fruit
Whole-grain bread
Coffee or tea

Design your own tossed seafood Louis. Combine a tossed lettuce salad with the shrimp or tuna and Jones Tomato Dressing. Garnish with tomato wedges. Another idea: Combine the seafood with a smaller amount of lettuce and finely chopped tomato and dressing and stuff it into whole-wheat pita bread for a pocket sandwich you can carry with you. You can make this type of salad-in-a-sandwich in a totally different range of flavors by combining lettuce and shrimp or tuna with chopped papaya and Jones Pineapple-Ginger Dressing for a tropical seafood-salad sandwich.

WEDNESDAY DINNER

Tossed salad (as much of any of the fresh greens
or vegetables on your Free-Food List as desired)
with lemon juice, vinegar or a Jones Dressing
1 broiled lamb chop, all visible fat removed, or
3 ounces sliced lean roast lamb
Brown rice, bulgur or baked potato
Steamed carrots or other colorful vegetable
1/2 cup non-fat milk or plain non-fat yogurt
Fresh pineapple or pineapple chunks packed in natural juice
Coffee or tea

Lamb happens to be my favorite red meat; unfortunately, however, I often don't like the lamb I am served in restaurants and other people's homes because it's overcooked and usually served with mint jelly. If you don't think you like lamb, it may very well be that you have never had lamb cooked medium-rare and served with a mustard sauce. Lamb Chops Dijon is probably the favorite dinner at the Canyon Ranch in Tucson, a vacation/fitness resort where we serve very little red meat and where I was told "not many people like lamb." Even if you don't want to take the time to use the rest of the Party Diet menu for this dinner (see page 72), try this recipe. If you don't have all the necessary ingredients, at least cook your lamb only until it is bright pink and serve it with Dijon-style mustard instead of mint jelly.

Try cooking your carrots in a small amount of chicken stock with a little crushed sweet basil or tarragon; or grate them and steam them until just crisp-tender and use your milk allowance to make the Curry Dip as a sauce for them. (This also makes a wonderful vegetarian entrée for lunch for Monday.) Your milk allowance could also be used for Breakfast Cheese on your baked potato. Use a little mint extract on your pineapple for dessert. (See recipe for Minted Pineapple.) With this menu I like to put Jones Tarragon Dressing on the salad.

THURSDAY

THURSDAY LUNCH

Raw vegetable relish tray or bag of vegetables
1/2 cup low-fat cottage cheese
or partially skimmed ricotta cheese or hoop cheese
Whole-grain bagel or whole-grain bread
Blueberries or available fresh fruit
Coffee or tea

This lunch is actually a duplicate of Monday's lunch only I specifically include bagels and blueberries. One of my favorite sandwiches is a combination of Breakfast Cheese and blueberries mixed together and spread on toasted pumpernickel bagel halves. At home, I serve the bagel open-faced and, if I am carrying them with me, I put the two halves back together with the blueberry mixture inside. You could combine the Breakfast Cheese with any fruit you like and carry a bag of raw vegetables for a well-balanced delicious lunch.

If you are at home, you might want to make a large vegetable salad, instead of a relish tray, with Jones Pineapple-Ginger Dressing, serving it with toasted whole-grain bread or bagels, and saving the blueberries for dessert, topped with Breakfast Cheese.

Still another possibility is to make Whole-Wheat Crêpes and fill them with one of the Mock Sour Cream Dips. I particularly like the Curry or Onion Dip as a filling. I serve an assortment of fresh fruit on the side—pineapple and melon are particularly good. When serving the onion crêpe, I like sliced apples.

You might want to substitute a baked potato for the bread, stuffing it with cottage cheese and chopped chives or green onion tops. Stuffed potatoes are also good cold for a brown bag lunch.

THURSDAY DINNER

Tossed salad (as much of any of the fresh greens
or vegetables on your Free-Food List as desired)
with lemon juice, vinegar or a Jones Dressing
1 baked or poached chicken breast without skin or
3 ounces white turkey meat without skin
Whole-wheat pasta, brown rice or bulgur
Brussels sprouts or available fresh green vegetable
Fresh peach, canned water-packed peach
or other available fresh fruit
1/2 cup non-fat milk or plain non-fat yogurt
Coffee or tea

Instead of having your bulgur as a hot side dish, use it to make Tabbouli, a wonderful Lebanese salad included in the recipe section, and
serve it with a broiled chicken breast. Cook the brussels sprouts in a
little chicken stock with caraway seeds. Sprinkle cinnamon on the
peach and place it under the broiler until it is hot and lightly browned;
then serve it either with plain yogurt or Yogurt Sauce.

FRIDAY

FRIDAY LUNCH

Raw vegetable relish tray or bag of vegetables
2 ounces hard cheese (American, cheddar, Jack, mozzarella, Swiss)
Corn tortilla or whole-wheat bread
Apple or available fresh fruit
Coffee or tea

Chop the raw vegetables and grate the cheese and add some shredded
lettuce, mixing all of it with a little Jones Tomato Dressing for a
sandwich on whole-wheat bread or in a pita pocket. Add an apple for
a brown bag lunch. I also like cheddar cheese and apple sandwiches. If
you are staying home, you may want to melt your cheese on a tortilla
or on bread for a melted cheese sandwich.

FRIDAY DINNER

Tossed salad (as much of any of the fresh greens
or vegetables on your Free-Food List as desired)
with lemon juice, vinegar or a Jones Dressing
4 ounces poached, broiled or baked fish or seafood
Pea pods or other green vegetable
Fresh pineapple or pineapple chunks canned in natural juice
1/2 cup non-fat milk or plain non-fat yogurt
Coffee or tea

Use your milk allowance to make Curry Dip for your salad dressing
and chop the pineapple into the salad. For a light supper in the summer,
you may also want to add cold chopped fish and cold steamed pea pods
to the salad. Cold brown rice would also go well in it. Or you may
want to serve the curried pineapple salad with broiled fish and rice or
bulgur mixed with chopped steamed vegetables.

SATURDAY

SATURDAY LUNCH

Raw vegetable relish tray or bag of vegetables
3 ounces crab, lobster or water-packed tuna or canned salmon
Whole-wheat lavash or whole-grain bread
Apple or available fresh fruit
1/2 cup non-fat milk or plain non-fat yogurt
Coffee or tea

Use your milk allowance to make the Dill Dip variation of the Mock
Sour Cream recipe and mix the salmon with the Dill Dip. Spread it on
pumpernickel bread for a truly delicious gourmet sandwich. You also
may want to add sliced cucumbers to this sandwich or put cucumber
sticks with your relish tray to go with the sandwich. Sprinkle the sliced
apple lightly with cinnamon and nutmeg for dessert. If you are at home
on Saturday, you may want to have a salad instead. Use the Dill Dip as
a salad dressing for a large tossed salmon, tuna or seafood salad and

serve it with whole-wheat lavash. If you use the dip for a salad, chop the apple up and add it also. It's a wonderful combination.

SATURDAY DINNER

Tossed salad (as much of any of the fresh greens
or vegetables on your Free-Food List as desired)
with lemon juice, vinegar or a Jones Dressing
3 ounces broiled steak, all visible fat removed
Baked potato
Steamed zucchini squash and onions
or available fresh green vegetable
Grapes or available fresh fruit
Coffee or tea

Use the Jones Cumin Dressing as a marinade for the steak. Toss the salad with the chunky variation of the Gazpacho and serve some of it as a sauce with the steak. Scoop out the baked potato and mix the pulp with the steamed vegetables (finely chopped). Cook them all in a little chicken stock and stuff back into the baked potato. Or combine the vegetables with brown rice to serve with the steak.

SUNDAY

SUNDAY LUNCH

Raw vegetable relish tray or bag of vegetables
1 egg, boiled, poached or cooked in a non-stick pan
1 ounce hard cheese (American, cheddar, Jack, mozzarella, Swiss)
Whole-wheat pita bread or other whole-grain bread
Melon or available fresh fruit
Coffee or tea

Hard cook the egg and chop finely. Shred the cheese and combine them both with an assortment of chopped raw or cold cooked vegetables and shredded lettuce or cabbage for a real chef's salad. Or use an additional egg *white* with the egg and make an omelet, using the grated cheese. Serve it with a tossed salad or relish tray and whole-grain toast.

Make a cantaloupe cooler, a refreshing beverage made with soda water and cantaloupe or other available melon. Combine them in a blender container, blend until smooth and pour over ice. You might want to use the egg raw for an egg nog or a smoothie. When using raw eggs or raw egg whites, it is important to coddle or dip the whole egg (in the shell) in boiling water for 30 seconds before using. This is because avedin, a component of raw egg whites, is believed to block the absorption of biotin, a water-soluble vitamin. Avedin is extremely sensitive to heat and coddling the egg inactivates it.

SUNDAY DINNER

Tossed salad (as much of any of the fresh greens
or vegetables on your Free-Food List as desired)
with lemon juice, vinegar or a Jones Dressing
3 ounces sliced white turkey meat without skin
Bulgur or brown rice
Beets or other colorful vegetable
Pear or available fresh fruit
1/2 cup non-fat milk or plain non-fat yogurt
Coffee or tea

Start with a salad with Jones Pineapple-Ginger Dressing, followed by turkey slices with Skinny Turkey Gravy and brown rice. I like the beets baked with a little chicken stock and caraway seeds. Serve the fruit plate with yogurt or Breakfast Cheese. Or if you want to make dinner ahead of time, make a turkey casserole by chopping up the turkey and cooked vegetables and adding brown rice or bulgur. Add a little chicken stock and bake, uncovered, until heated through.

Party
Weight-Loss Diet

If you are a food lover who wishes to cook more elaborate meals than those offered on the Basic Weight-Loss Diet, the Party Diet may be used as a total or partial replacement. Although the Party Diet is specifically designed for entertaining or other special occasions while on the Basic Weight-Loss Diet, it can be substituted whenever you wish.

MONDAY

MONDAY LUNCH

Tossed green salad with Jones Italian Dressing
Pasta Primavera
Fresh Fruit Compote
Coffee or tea

Have an interesting pasta buffet. Steam all of the vegetables separately and have them in individual bowls surrounding the pasta. Each guest can add the vegetable he likes best and design his own Pasta Primavera. Or if you are serving individually, serve the pasta and pass bowls of the different vegetables, just as you would pass condiments for curry.

MONDAY DINNER

Raw vegetable relish tray with 2 tablespoons Jones Dip
Poached Bass in Dill Sauce
Wild Rice Pilaf
Herbed Carrots
Banana Sorbet
Coffee or tea

This dinner can be turned into a beautiful buffet by using an assortment of raw vegetables cut into interesting shapes to garnish the Poached Bass in Dill Sauce. Also, the bass and vegetables can be served either hot or cold. The Herbed Carrots can be turned into herbed carrot flowers. There are several good books on garniture that will teach you to make flowers and other interesting designs out of fruits and vegetables. If you are serving this dinner buffet style, put only the entrée out for buffet service and serve the Banana Sorbet to your guests individually. It is not a practical dessert for a buffet because it melts!

TUESDAY

TUESDAY LUNCH

Raw vegetable relish tray with 2 tablespoons Jones Dip
Baked Tuna in Tomato Bowl
Whole-grain rolls
Strawberries Romanoff
Coffee or tea

This lunch makes a beautiful plate if the vegetables are used for garniture. Remember—visual pleasure must always be considered when planning a menu. This is also a wonderful lunch to make ahead of time. Everything except the last-minute preparations can be done a day in advance. The Baked Tuna in Tomato Bowl is also wonderful as a leftover, served cold.

TUESDAY DINNER

Tossed salad (as much of any of the fresh greens
or vegetables on your Free-Food List as desired)
with Jones Pineapple-Ginger Dressing
Lemon Chicken in Envelopes
Lemon Onion Bulgur
Steamed broccoli
Mediterranean Melon Balls
Coffee or tea

This is a tasty Middle Eastern party menu. Garnish plates with grape leaves and add cinnamon to your coffee or tea with dessert. If you really want to go all the way with the Middle Eastern motif, hire a belly dancer to entertain your guests after dinner—or better yet, take belly dancing lessons and perform yourself! It's a great aerobic exercise.

WEDNESDAY

WEDNESDAY LUNCH

Raw vegetable relish tray
Curried Shrimp or Crab in Papaya Cups
Whole-wheat matzos
Coffee or tea

This menu makes an elegant one-plate luncheon. Serve the papaya cup surrounded by a colorful assortment of other fruits and vegetables with whole-wheat matzo on the side. This is a very practical menu for a large buffet where guests have to balance plates on their knees. You only need one utensil—a fork—and, because your fruit, vegetable and protein are all served at the same time, you do not have to worry about collecting plates and replacing them between courses.

WEDNESDAY DINNER

Fresh mushroom and watercress salad with Jones Tarragon Dressing
1 Lamb Chop Dijon
Stuffed Baked Potato
Herbed Carrots
Minted Pineapple
Coffee or tea

This menu is perfect for company because all the dishes can be prepared in advance. You can cook the lamb chops and then reheat the stuffed baked potatoes and herbed carrots in a half hour. While the lamb chops are cooking, you can toss the salad, put it on chilled plates and bring it to the table. Garnish the Minted Pineapple with sprigs of fresh mint, if available.

THURSDAY

THURSDAY LUNCH

Raw vegetable relish tray
2 Crêpes Florentine
Tomato Provençal
Fresh blueberries
Coffee or tea

This luncheon menu also works well for brunch. When serving it for brunch, you might have a first course of Blueberry Soup instead of serving fresh blueberries for dessert; garnish the entrée plate with the raw vegetables and skip the relish tray.

THURSDAY DINNER

Stracciatelle alla Romana
Tossed salad (as much of any of the fresh greens
or vegetables on your Free-Food List as desired)
with Jones Italian Dressing

Fettuccine Cacciatore
Herbed Vegetable Medley
Peaches "Amaretto"
Coffee or tea

A perfect menu for an Italian dinner party. Parties are more fun and easier to plan when you have a theme. Your invitations and decor, as well as the menu, should reflect your theme. For an Italian dinner you might send invitations with Italian flags or drawings of gondolas on them. Use a checkered tablecloth similar to those used in many Italian restaurants and raffia-wrapped Italian wine bottles for candleholders.

FRIDAY

FRIDAY LUNCH

Gazpacho
Tostada
Baked Apple
Coffee or tea

This Mexican menu is another good theme-party idea. The last time I served it, I put little Mexican flags on top of all the Tostadas. Place mats and napkins in a variety of bright colors work well for a Mexican motif. Hiring a mariachi band is wonderful too—but not essential—recordings and tapes are also available.

FRIDAY DINNER

Egg Flower Soup
Seafood Chow Mein
Brown rice
Pineapple Boats with Coconut Sauce
Tea

This Chinese party menu can be lots of fun. Give chopsticks to all of your guests, along with forks wrapped in the napkins—just in case!

Instead of fortune cookies, type out your own fortunes for each of your guests and wrap them around cinnamon sticks. Put a cinnamon stick in each Pineapple Boat.

SATURDAY

SATURDAY LUNCH

Sherried Consommé
Curried Seafood Salad
Whole-wheat lavash
Coffee or tea

This menu works well when you are entertaining for lunch. Try it the next time you are having your bridge group or a group from the office over. Everything can be prepared ahead of time and combined just before serving. Because there is fresh fruit in the salad, a dessert is unnecessary.

SATURDAY DINNER

Tossed salad (as much of any of the fresh greens
or vegetables on your Free-Food List as desired)
with Jones Tomato Dressing
Teriyaki Steak
Overbaked Potato
Herbed Zucchini and Onions
Sherried Grapes
Coffee or tea

This menu works wonderfully for an outdoor barbecue. I always like to use paper products for outdoor cooking; it's so nice to be able to clean up by putting your tablecloth or mats and napkins all in the wastebasket. You can go one step further and use paper plates too! A backyard barbecue can be as informal or as elegant as you wish to make it. You can light your outdoor area with flaming tiki torches or hang Chinese lanterns.

SUNDAY

SUNDAY LUNCH

Fake Margarita
Raw vegetable relish tray with 2 tablespoons Jones Mexican Dip
Huevos Rancheros
Mexican fruit plate
(This is a colorful combination of all fruits grown in Mexico;
since all fruits are grown in Mexico, a colorful combination
of whatever is available constitutes a "Mexican fruit plate.")
Coffee or tea

This menu is great for a Mexican brunch. It can also be fun for birthday parties. Pinatas, so perfect for Mexican fiestas, are usually filled with candy. Fill yours with gag gifts for all of your friends. Or if you are entertaining bankers, fill it with money!

SUNDAY DINNER

Asparagus Vinaigrette
Coq au Vin
Rice Pilaf
Beets seasoned with dill
Poached Pear in Sauterne Sauce
Coffee or tea

I like to use this menu for a French dinner party, giving each guest a copy of the menu in French:

ASPERGES VINAIGRETTE

COQ AU VIN

RIZ PILAF

BETTERAVES À L'ANETH

POIRE AU SAUTERNE

CAFÉ OU THÉ

PERRIER '82

Vegetarian Weight-Loss Diet

If you are a vegetarian, you may use the Vegetarian Diet to replace the Basic Weight-Loss Diet. Many of the meals are identical to those on the Basic Diet. For ideas on how to add variety to each meal, read the suggestions I have included with the daily menus in the section on the Basic Weight-Loss Diet. Even if you are not a vegetarian, you may find that many of the vegetarian entrées listed make delicious and economical alternative meals.

VEGETARIANISM

The most complete definition of vegetarianism that I have read appears in the *Vegetarian Voice:* "Abstinence from meat, fish and fowl with or without the use of dairy products or eggs. Consisting primarily of plant foods such as beans, grains, fruits, vegetables, seed and nuts, the vegetarian diet closely resembles the original human diet. Lacto-vegetarians use dairy products; ovo-vegetarians use eggs; lacto-ovo-vegetarians use both. Total vegetarians and vegans consume no food of animal origin, including dairy products and eggs."

Providing sufficient protein for the growth, maintenance and repair of body cells in a vegan-vegetarian diet involves the principle of protein complementarity. The word "complement" is defined as "providing something that is lacking or needed." To vegetarians of all persuasions, *complementarity* is a key word. Protein complementarity is the pairing of essential amino acids.

Proteins are made of 22 amino acids, nine of which must be obtained from the food we eat. These nine amino acids are called the

76

essential amino acids. They include histidine, isoleucine, leucine, lysine, methionine, phenylalanine, threonine, tryptophan and valine. Animal proteins are considered to be of higher quality than plant proteins because they are composed of all the essential amino acids (the building blocks of protein) in the proportions in which the body can best use them. All plant proteins lack one or more of the essential amino acids; however, combinations or pairing of plant proteins in your daily diet give about the same nutritional value as good quality animal proteins.

In complementing the proteins to obtain the most usable protein for the body, it is necessary to combine a plant food with weak amino acids with another food which is high in those amino acids and thus make up for the deficiency. For example, rice is low in lysine but when eaten with dried beans the beans provide the needed lysine. By the same token, rice supplies methionine, which is in short supply in the bean protein. Three-quarters cup of beans combined (or eaten at the same meal) with two cups of rice provides approximately the same amount of usable protein as found in a six-ounce steak.

The following chart shows the basic combinations of food involved in the complementing process:

PROTEIN COMPLEMENTARITY

	GRAINS	MILK PRODUCTS	SEEDS
LEGUMES	XX	X	XX
MILK PRODUCTS	XX		
SEEDS	X	X	

XX   Most combinations will form complete protein
 X   A few combinations will form complete protein

Strict vegetarian diets are deficient in Vitamin B-12. It is also difficult to get enough calcium without dairy products, and Vitamin D is usually found in enriched milk. Strict vegetarianism is considered dangerous by many physicians for growing children, pregnant women and nursing mothers. However, these dangers do not exist for lacto-ovo-vegetarians. Dairy products and eggs contain an excellent balance of the essential amino acids, and they combine with lower quality proteins in plant food, making them complete proteins as well. For these reasons the Food Lover's Vegetarian Diet includes both dairy products and eggs.

BREAKFAST

1/2 grapefruit or 1 orange
(fresh fruit not juice)
Whole-grain bread or whole-grain cereal
1/2 cup non-fat milk or plain non-fat yogurt;
or 1/4 cup low-fat cottage cheese,
hoop cheese or partially skimmed ricotta cheese
Coffee or tea

MONDAY

LUNCH

Raw vegetable relish tray or bag of vegetables
1/2 cup low-fat cottage cheese, hoop cheese
or partially skimmed ricotta cheese
Fresh fruit
Whole-grain bread or whole-grain pasta
Coffee or tea

DINNER

Tossed salad (as much of any of the fresh greens
or vegetables on your Free-Food List as desired)
with lemon juice, vinegar or a Jones Dressing
Tamale Pie
Steamed vegetables (colorful assortment)
Banana or available fresh fruit
1/2 cup non-fat milk or plain non-fat yogurt
Coffee or tea

TUESDAY

LUNCH

Raw vegetable relish tray or bag of vegetables
Stuffed Tomato Bowls
Whole-grain bread
Strawberries or available fresh fruit
1/2 cup non-fat milk or plain non-fat yogurt
Coffee or tea

DINNER

Tossed salad (as much of any of the fresh greens
or vegetables on your Free-Food List as desired)
with lemon juice, vinegar or a Jones Dressing
Vegetarian Lasagna
Steamed vegetable
Melon or available fresh fruit
Coffee or tea

WEDNESDAY

LUNCH

Raw vegetable relish tray or bag of vegetables
Curried Tofu and Pineapple Salad
Whole-grain bread
Coffee or tea

DINNER

Tossed salad (as much of any of the fresh greens
or vegetables on your Free-Food List as desired)
with lemon juice, vinegar or a Jones Dressing
East Indian Carrot Casserole
Brown rice or bulgur
Steamed vegetable
1/2 cup non-fat milk or plain non-fat yogurt
Fresh pineapple or pineapple chunks packed in natural juice
Coffee or tea

THURSDAY

LUNCH

Raw vegetable relish tray or bag of vegetables
1/2 cup low-fat cottage cheese
or partially skimmed ricotta cheese or hoop cheese
Whole-grain bagel or whole-grain bread
Blueberries or available fresh fruit
Coffee or tea

DINNER

Tossed salad (as much of any of the fresh greens
or vegetables on your Free-Food List as desired)
with lemon juice, vinegar or a Jones Dressing

Vegetarian Fettuccine Cacciatore
Steamed vegetable
Fresh peach or canned water-packed peach or available fresh fruit
1/2 cup non-fat milk or plain non-fat yogurt
Coffee or tea

FRIDAY

LUNCH

Raw vegetable relish tray or bag of vegetables
2 ounces hard cheese (American, cheddar, Jack, mozzarella, Swiss)
Corn tortilla or whole-wheat bread
Apple or available fresh fruit
Coffee or tea

DINNER

Tossed salad (as much of any of the fresh greens
or vegetables on your Free-Food List as desired)
with lemon juice, vinegar or a Jones Dressing
Tofu Vegetarian Chow Mein
Brown rice or bulgur
Fresh pineapple or pineapple chunks canned in natural juice
1/2 cup non-fat milk or plain non-fat yogurt
Coffee or tea

SATURDAY

LUNCH

Raw vegetable relish tray or bag of vegetables
2 Crêpes Florentine
Apple or available fresh fruit
1/2 cup non-fat milk or plain non-fat yogurt
Coffee or tea

DINNER

Tossed salad (as much of any of the fresh greens
or vegetables on your Free-Food List as desired)
with lemon juice, vinegar or a Jones Dressing
Vegetarian White Chili
Steamed zucchini squash and onions or available fresh green vegetable
Frozen Grapes or available fresh fruit
Coffee or tea

SUNDAY

LUNCH

Raw vegetable relish tray or bag of vegetables
1 egg, boiled, poached or cooked in a non-stick pan
1 ounce hard cheese (American, cheddar, Jack, mozzarella, Swiss)
Whole-wheat pita bread or other whole-grain bread
Melon or available fresh fruit
Coffee or tea

DINNER

Tossed salad (as much of any of the fresh greens
or vegetables on your Free-Food List as desired)
with lemon juice, vinegar or a Jones Dressing
Lentils au Gratin
Beets or other colorful vegetable
Pear or available fresh fruit
1/2 cup non-fat milk or plain non-fat yogurt
Coffee or tea

Lifetime Diet

The motto of the Food Lover's Lifetime dieters is *never say never!* You can eat or drink anything you want because you have learned *how.* After finishing this book you will have learned all of the basics of good nutrition. You will know *what* is important in a good lifetime diet program and you will know *why.*

You are now ready to start planning your own diet. You can use the other diet menus in this book as guidelines, with complete freedom to add salad dressings, sauces and your favorite desserts wherever you wish, remembering that the rules of good nutrition still apply and that moderation and common sense are the two most important dietary laws. The Food Lists at the back of the book show practically every known food, including many things which are *not* recommended for good nutrition; but since they do exist and are no longer strictly off limits to you, I am providing the nutritional information you may want to know.

ADDING FAT AND ALCOHOL TO YOUR DIET

When adding fat to your diet, start slowly and stop before the additions are significant. For example, if you are having Eggs Benedict for brunch, don't order Beef Stroganoff for dinner. If you want a Ramos Fizz, ask the bartender to make it with milk instead of cream. If you are going to a wine and food society dinner in the evening, don't stay home the night before and put butter and sour cream on your potato. Remember—you aren't after a *fat attack,* but rather the latitude and freedom to enjoy the wonderful culinary creations you love—in reasonable amounts—which means continuing to apply the laws of common sense and moderation.

When adding alcohol to your diet, try to limit yourself to two drinks a day. If you want to have wine with dinner, it is best to forego cocktails before the meal. Conversely, if you would like to have a cocktail or two before dinner, it's best to pass on the wine. Also, do not order distilled spirits "on the rocks" but with water or soda. You can extend the calories in wine by ordering wine spritzers where the wine is served with ice and soda water. When ordering beer, or buying beer, choose one of the light low-calorie varieties.

PLANNING YOUR LIFETIME DIET

I should point out that the word "diet" is perhaps one of the most misused words in the English language. It is not something you "go on" and then "go off." According to Webster, diet is "food and drink regularly provided or consumed—habitual course of feeding." In other words, you are *always* on a diet; whether it's a good diet or a bad diet is up to you. Think of your Lifetime Diet as a permanent, studied change in your life-style. You may still make mistakes and eat or drink too much of the wrong things, but you now know how easy it is to get right back on the track.

The food requirements I am giving for a well-balanced diet at 1500 calories per day leave all of the choices up to you (see the Food Lists in the appendix for information you need to make your selections). Use the charts I have included to keep a record of all the nutritional information about your daily menu plans. To help you in completing the chart and give you menu ideas at two different calorie levels, I have filled in two charts as examples. There is also an example of how to break down recipes into food groups to determine their calories and food group portions, as well as the cholesterol and sodium content. Note that there are a number of ingredients, such as fat-free stock, herbs and spices and all the raw vegetables on the Free-Food List, in which the calories are negligible and need not be counted. With this information you can determine the number of calories per serving in your favorite recipes and perhaps lower the calories considerably by using the information in Helpful Hints and Honest Cheating.

After you start your own Lifetime Diet, weigh yourself weekly. Any time your weight starts back up, quickly apply the Diet Brakes described in detail in the following chapter. Don't ever wait to hit the brakes. The sooner you do it, the easier it is to *stop*. Now, start planning your menus and organizing your parties on a diet plan you can stay on safely forever. Bon appétit!

The following guidelines for diets at the 1500 and 2500 calorie per day levels are easy to follow if you use the Food Lists to plan your menus. A sample menu at each calorie level has been written on the following charts. There is also a blank chart for you to use as a sample in making your own charts.

1500 CALORIES PER DAY	2500 CALORIES PER DAY
4 fruit portions	6 fruit portions
6–8 starch portions	10–15 vegetable portions
6–8 vegetable portions	10–15 starch portions
6 protein portions (low fat when possible)	6 protein portions (low fat when possible)
4 fat portions	6 fat portions
2 milk portions (non-fat when possible)	2 milk portions (non-fat when possible)

I suggest planning your meals ahead of time rather than just keeping records of what you eat. This allows you to exchange one food for another that is lower in sodium or cholesterol within the same group. For instance, if your projected sodium figure for a given day is well over 2000 milligrams, look carefully at each meal to see what items can be replaced with foods containing less sodium. Instead of having one-half cup of Grapenuts cereal for breakfast, which contains 294 milligrams of sodium, you might substitute a large shredded wheat biscuit, which has one milligram of sodium. If you had planned to have one-half cup of cottage cheese for lunch, which contains 468 milligrams of sodium, you could exchange it for two ounces of chicken, which constains only 44 milligrams of sodium. As I said before, the options are limitless. You can really have fun learning while you lose!

DAY _____		PORTIONS										SUMMARY					
					Protein				Milk								
		Fruit	Vegetables	Starch	L	M	H	Fat	N	L	W	Calories	Carbohydrates	Protein	Fat	Mg. Cholesterol	Mg. Sodium
B R E A K F A S T																	
L U N C H																	
D I N N E R																	
Totals																	

				PORTIONS								SUMMARY					
					Protein				Milk								
DAY _Tuesday_		Fruit	Vegetables	Starch	L	M	H	Fat	N	L	W	Calories	Carbohydrates	Protein	Fat	Mg. Cholesterol	Mg. Sodium
1500 Calories approx.																	
B R E A K F A S T	½ grapefruit	1										40	10				1
	1 c. 7 grain cereal			2								140	30	4			2
	¾ c. nonfat milk								¾			60	9	6		.7	95
	½ banana	1										40	10				.5
L U N C H	chicken salad w/ peapods and				2							110		14	6	50	44
	water chestnuts		4									100	20	8			16
																	16A
	¼ c. jones dressing			3								210	45	6			399
	1½ english muffin w/ 1 tbl. corn oil margarine							3				135			15		105
	cheesecake - 2 portions	1			1			1				140	10	7	8	186	276
	½ c. non-fat milk								½			40	6	4		.2	6A
D I N N E R	1 sliced tomato		1									25	5	2			6
	3 oz. salmon, poached				3							165		21	9	55	42
	1 lrg. baked potato w/			2								140	30	4			4
	¼ c. mustard dip							¼				20	3	2		4	29
	½ c. carrots		1									25	5	2	2		24
	1 c. asparagus		1									25	5	2			1
	¾ c. strawberries	1										40	10				1
	w/ ½ c. non-fat milk								½			40	6	4		1.2	6A
Totals		4	7	7	6			4	2			1495	205	86	40	1319	1337.5

				PORTIONS						SUMMARY							
					Protein				Milk								
DAY Thursday / 2500 Calories approx.		Fruit	Vegetables	Starch	L	M	H	Fat	N	L	W	Calories	Carbohydrates	Protein	Fat	Mg. Cholesterol	Mg. Sodium
BREAKFAST	1 sliced orange	1										40	10				1
	1½ c. oatmeal			3								210	45	6			3
	1 c. non-fat milk								1			80	12	8		2.3	127
	¾ c. strawberries	1										40	10				1
	2 slices whole wheat toast w/			2								140	30	4			272
	1 tbl. corn oil margarine							3				135			15		105
	4 tbls. apple butter	1										40	10				1
LUNCH	wedge of cantaloupe (2 servings of)	2										80	20				20
	pasta primavera w/		4	2				½				278	50	16	3	7.4	28
	½ c. lowfat cottage cheese					2						110				5.2	468
	1 whole grain roll w/			1								70	15	2			143
	¼ tsp. corn oil margarine							¼				12			2		9
	½ c. non-fat milk								½			40	6	4		1.2	64
	jelled fruitcake	1						¼				52	10		2		12
DINNER	vegetable salad w/		2									50	10	4			20
	oil and vinegar dressing							¾				36			4		82
	4 oz. steak						4					220		28	12	120	68
	2 c. brown rice			6								420	90	12			36
	½ c. sweet potato			2								140	30	4			14
	1 c. broccoli		1									25	5	2			22
	1 baked onion		2									50	10	4			18
	½ c. non-fat milk								½			40	6	4		1.2	64
	holiday pumpkin cream			¼	½							66	4	4	2	5	13
Totals		6	9	16¼	6½	½		4¼	2			2374	373	102	40	423	1591

CALCULATING RECIPES

I included my own notes with the following recipe to show how to calculate the nutritional information for your own recipes. Check each ingredient on the Food Lists, making sure that you have the right food group listed and the correct number of portions listed for it so that calories and food group portions will be accurate. Remember that within each food group amounts equalling one portion will vary. For example, one cup of broccoli equals one Vegetable Portion, but one-half cup of carrots equals one Vegetable Portion, and only one-quarter cup of peas equals one Vegetable Portion. If you had one cup of peas you would have eaten four Vegetable Portions; similarly, one cup of carrots would equal two Vegetable Portions. One cup of orange juice equals two Fruit Portions; however, one cup of grape juice equals four Fruit Portions.

Cholesterol	Sodium	TOSTADA	
	TR	4 tortillas, toasted (whole or in tortilla chips)	4 starches 280 Cal
	42	1 head lettuce, finely chopped	free food
	12	2 medium tomatoes, diced	2 vegetables 50 Cal.
	328	1/2 cup Jones Cumin Dressing, page 128-129	
154.8	132	1-1/2 cups chicken or turkey, cooked and diced	6 low-fat proteins 330 Cal
60.2	386	1/2 cup grated cheddar or Monterey Jack cheese	2 high-fat proteins 190 cal
2.9	243	1/4 cup Mock Sour Cream, page 133	1 low-fat protein 55 cal.
		Chopped tomatoes for garnish	905 cal.
217.9	1143		

Makes 4 servings
Each serving contains approximately:
1 starch portion 70
1/2 vegetable portion 13
1 3/4 low-fat protein portions 96
1/2 high-fat protein portion 48
227 calories
55 mg. cholesterol
286 mg. sodium

DIET BRAKES

When using the Food Lover's Diet, think of the food groups or calorie sources as traffic lights on a three-light signal. The green light on the top means *go,* or unlimited eating; and the red light at the bottom means *stop*—not allowed at all. The green light represents complex carbohydrates, which are unlimited on both the Basic Diet and the Lifetime Diet. The yellow light represents animal protein and refined carbohydrates, which are limited on both the Basic Diet and the Lifetime Diet. The red light represents added fats and alcohol which are *not* allowed on the Basic Diet and are limited on the Lifetime Diet.

Just as you can mix and match the meals on the Basic Diet and Party Diet, even parts of meals if you wish, you can also go back and forth between the Basic Diet and the Lifetime Diet from day to day or meal to meal. This is what I call *applying the diet brakes.* Remember the signal on the Basic Weight-Loss Diet is always red for added fat and alcohol. The Lifetime Diet signal does not have a red light, though it does turn yellow to control the amounts of fat and alcohol, along with animal protein and refined carbohydrates, that you consume. Whenever you start to gain weight, the red light is again in effect. Just apply the brakes, cutting out added fat and alcohol until you are back to your desired weight. Or you can tailor your braking program to fit into your own life-style.

If you are going to a party where you will want a glass of wine or a mixed drink instead of limiting yourself to soda water all evening, carefully watch your fat intake and trim your portion sizes during the rest of the day. Then go to the party, have a drink, enjoy your dinner and return home happy—*not* guilty. In other words, you can eat and drink anything you want once you have learned *how.* This is an educational program built into a diet. After reading this book and following the Food Lover's Weight-Loss Diets for two weeks, you have an understanding of nutrition and the behavioral patterns needed to live better for the rest of your life.

The problem with most diet books is that they tell you *what* to do—without ever telling you *why.* These diets also lack variety, so people get bored eating the same foods every day. When their enthusiasm wears thin—and it always does—they have not acquired the knowledge necessary to help themselves and they go right back to the diet pattern that got them into trouble in the first place.

With the Food Lover's Diet, the days of the "yo-yo syndrome"—losing weight this week only to gain it back the next—are over forever for you. After being on this diet for two weeks you can't help but feel better, look better and have more energy than you have had in a long time. You may even feel smarter and find your memory has improved—the brain is an organ like any other and it responds favorably to good nutrition. You are not likely to give up on a diet program that contributes so dramatically to your sense of well-being, self-confidence and happiness—especially when you know better!

HOW TO STOP LOSING WEIGHT

Many people find that after reaching their desired weight on the Food Lover's Diet they go right on losing more weight. This is generally because the combination of foods is such that the body works more efficiently and it takes more calories to maintain the same weight. However, to gain weight, you certainly do not want to start eating fatty junk foods or ultimately you will be right back where you started—fat and miserable!

I was appalled by the advice of a physician on gaining weight that appeared in a recently published, popular diet book. He suggested adding high-calorie snacks such as sweets, potato chips and nuts throughout the day and evening. He also recommended not trimming fat from meat or removing skin from poultry, and then covering them with rich sauces and gravies; eating buttered breads and biscuits, pies and cakes; and always choosing fruits canned in heavy syrups. Other desserts included ice cream sundaes with fudge and butterscotch sauces and thick puddings topped with whipped cream. For breakfast, he suggested loading cereals with cream and sugar. Beverages included ice cream sodas, thick milk shakes, malteds, whole milk, chocolate milk and heavy cream and sugar in hot chocolate, coffee and tea.

A desire to gain weight does *not* mean that you want to increase your chances of heart disease and general lack of fitness. Therefore, the same principles of good nutrition apply to gaining weight that apply to losing and maintaining weight. The green light for *go,* or unlimited eating, still only holds for complex carbohydrates. Fat, alcohol and animal proteins remain limited. The secret to reversing the weight-loss cycle, maintaining a desired weight or returning to a desired weight is to increase with moderation the portion sizes of the complex carbohydrates and polyunsaturated fats and to increase how often you eat. Add a midmorning, midafternoon and bedtime snack to your diet. Even if you work you can carry rolls, bagels or a baked potato with you in a bag. You may also want to add more fruit to your diet. Bananas are ideal fruits to carry with you because they grow their own wrappings—just peel and eat!

If you continue to lose weight after starting to eat more and more frequently, consult your doctor. The weight loss may be caused by a medical problem of which you aren't aware.

Life-Style

This section of the book deals with many of the important facets of your life that are food related—things that are important for everyone to be aware of and *essential* for the food lover who wants to maintain a desired weight.

SPECIAL OCCASIONS:
(THE EXCEPTIONS TO THE RULES)

Special occasions, including religious holidays such as Christmas, Hanukkah, Passover and Easter, national holidays such as Thanksgiving Day, Memorial Day and the Fourth of July, as well as birthdays, graduations, christenings, Bar and Bat Mitzvahs, weddings, anniversaries, etc., are often used as excuses to overeat and overdrink. If you make all these special occasions exceptions, you will quickly find it is possible to make exceptions to the rules out of almost 365 days a year.

Almost all religious holidays are either fast days or feast days. And yet have you ever stopped to realize how much media attention fast days receive versus feast days? It is about one hundred to zero in favor of feasts! Along with each of these feast days come traditional foods. In the food sense, "tradition" equals high calorie density; however, it is not usually necessary to add all of the fat and refined carbohydrates called for in "traditional" holiday recipes. In fact, most of these traditional foods are better when prepared with less fat and sugar and refined flours are replaced with their whole-grain counterparts.

For example, the Wild Rice Pilaf (or the Brown Rice Pilaf) recipe in this book is excellent served as a dressing with holiday turkey. Fruit Compote is delicious served for dessert on the same menu, replacing the more traditional, super-rich fruit cake or plum pudding. The Holiday Pumpkin Cream and the Jelled Fruit Cake (in the recipe section) are other wonderful holiday desserts for food lovers who want to look terrific *after* the holidays too.

The most visually beautiful birthday dessert I have ever served was a large, round serving platter covered with Pineapple Boats in Coconut Sauce (see recipe). I arranged the pineapple quarters so that the leafy top portions were all on the outside of the platter, forming a green wreath. Then I placed birthday candles in the centers of the pineapple boats and lit them before carrying the tray to the table. It was such a tremendous hit that I have since served it for numerous birthday parties.

Special occasions are not the only time many people knowingly overeat foods that are not good for them. There are also many *daily* exceptions to the rules. Take, for example, the secretary who started a new diet program on Monday. A friend in the office brought in homemade cookies, and she couldn't very well hurt her friend's feelings by not eating one—but of course this was an exception to her diet rules, which wouldn't happen again. Until the office party the next day for the boss's birthday, that is; the birthday cake served was another necessary exception. Or perhaps you hadn't planned to drink any wine with dinner but the host poured a fabulous French Bordeaux wine you couldn't resist—again, it was an *exception*. Unfortunately, most of the foods and beverages which fall into the "exceptions" category also fall into the high-calorie-density category and are also usually low in nutritive density.

Between-meal goodies are common "exceptions." Goodies are foods that contain sugar, fat or salt, and often all three. Goodies are things like candy bars, cookies, salted nuts, potato and corn chips, ice cream cones and the like. People who are compulsive goodie-eaters have come by the habit honestly I assure you. Most children are taught early in life that goodies are comforting and solve all sorts of problems.

When a little boy who is just learning to walk falls down and skins his knee, have you ever seen a parent go running to him with a carrot stick to make him feel better? Of course not. It's usually a cookie or a piece of candy that is supposed to make his hurt "all better." Unfortunately, even after we know where these bad habits start, they are often still difficult to break. But remember the old cliché: "Eat it today— wear it tomorrow." Now that you are an adult a carrot stick will probably look a lot better on you than a cookie—even if you have skinned your knee!

ENTERTAINING—WITH A FLAIR AND A CONSCIENCE

Entertaining seems to be the real Achilles heel for most calorie-con- scious hosts and hostesses. For some reason the word "company" has come to mean "to kill." You may routinely serve your own family simple, low-calorie dinners such as a salad with a light dressing, broiled fish or chicken, a baked potato, some steamed vegetables and fresh fruit for dessert. But the minute you are planning for "company" the whole concept of eating changes. You certainly couldn't serve "com- pany" a light, low-calorie dinner for fear of insulting them. So you whip up a bleu cheese dressing to add hundreds of calories and grams of fat to the salad; sauté the chicken in butter; make a rice pilaf with still more butter; pour hollandaise sauce over the vegetables; and turn the fresh fruit into a pie with a flaky butter crust and lots of sugar in the fruit; and then if the "company" is *really* important, you serve the pie à la mode! In fact, it seems the more important the company is, the harder you try to kill them.

This philosophy of entertaining isn't just observed at dinner either. Long before dinner is put on the table, you serve cocktails with hors d'oeuvre, and certainly not your usual selection of raw or blanched vegetables with a low-calorie dip. For company, you serve a "real," high-calorie dip with chips, rumake, quiche or some other calorie- loaded hors d'oeuvre. After the meal, you serve coffee with brandy or liqueurs and pass after-dinner mints and nuts. Another thing you probably do for your "company" is serve portions twice the size you normally serve your own family. You certainly wouldn't want your guests to think you were being stingy with the food. To top it off, you watch them carefully to see how much they eat, ensuring feelings of guilt on the part of those who don't eat "appreciatively"!

The next time you plan a dinner party, think of this syndrome as a coin with two sides. One side says "company" and the other side says "guest," which is what you are when you are someone's "company."

Wouldn't you rather go to dinner in someone's home without feeling that you have to eat practically nothing for a day before or go on a rigid weight-loss program for two days after in order to maintain your weight? Wouldn't it be more fun to know you are going to get a light, delicious and imaginative meal served in reasonable amounts? Then you could thoroughly enjoy being a guest, experiencing no guilt for your own overindulgence or for hurting the feelings of your host or hostess, and you could leave with that wonderful feeling of having dined well *and* intelligently.

Even though you love food, there are lots of other things in life— none of them is fun or exciting when you're too full. Whether you are entertaining, being entertained or eating alone, think back to the last time you pushed yourself away from the table miserably uncomfortable. Let your imagination run wild. You can't think of one single thing you felt like doing except sitting down in a comfortable spot and waiting until that stuffed, miserable feeling passed. Food abuse, like drug abuse, leaves you incapacitated.

When planning your next party menu, use the Food Lover's Party Diet menus as a guide. All of the menus have been designed around a theme. For instance, the Italian dinner of Fettuccine Cacciatore starts with Stracciatelle alla Romana, a light Roman soup, the salad has an Italian dressing and Peaches "Amaretto" is a decidedly Italian dessert. If serving wine, you might select an Italian Soave, a dry white wine, to go with your Italian dinner. You may want to add a higher calorie dish or two to a Food Lover's Party Diet menu, using the guidelines for the Lifetime Diet, on which everything is allowed, but in moderation. You do not want every course of a meal to be a rich, high-calorie dish or, instead of ending up with a perfectly balanced gourmet meal, you will have a debauchery. Culinary creativity is not limited by anything but your own imagination. And remember that entertaining is far more than the food you serve. Entertaining is the ambiance you create with your table setting, flower arrangement or other unusual centerpiece you use. Even lighting is important. You will find out how quickly you can become the most popular host or hostess in your community with this new approach to entertaining—with a *flair and a conscience.*

Shopping and cooking for entertaining should be no more work and even more fun than your day-to-day food preparation. When possible, start preparing for a dinner party at least three days in advance. Make your shopping list and shop for everything you can, excluding perishable items which must be purchased on the day of the party. When you are shopping in a supermarket, always shop the walls—that's where you will find all of your basic, unprocessed foods. On one wall, you will find fresh fruits and vegetables; on another wall, you will find fresh fish, poultry and meat and essential dairy products, such as milk, yogurt and cottage cheese; and basic bakery goods, such as bread and rolls, are usually on yet another wall. What does that leave in the middle? All of the junk—the processed foods for which you are not only paying an exorbitant price, but which contain more fat, more salt, more refined sugar and more preservatives than the unprocessed equivalents. There are a few things in the middle aisles that you will need: powdered and canned milk, cereals, pasta, beans, herbs and spices and some frozen and canned goods. And, of course, cleaning products, paper goods, pet food, drug items, etc. Make your shopping list so that all of the items in the middle of the market are on top. Then once you have picked them up—get out—back to the walls and to your serious shopping.

This method of shopping also saves lots of money because it keeps you from browsing and buying things on impulse that you don't need.

When making your shopping list, it is also a good idea to write simply "fresh fruit" and "fresh vegetables." Choose your fruit and vegetables according to which ones look best in the market. Fresh produce "in season" is always the best buy. It is the best tasting, best looking *and* least expensive. So unless you are set on having midwinter fresh peaches flown in from New Zealand, wait until you are in the produce department to make your final decisions.

When you are cooking for a party—or any other time—always wear tight-fitting clothes. Tight jeans are ideal. Do *not* wear loose-fitting caftans or a sloppy over-sized shirt and pants, or you will eventually grow to fit them! Wearing tight clothing that makes you consciously stand up straight and hold your stomach in to be comfortable, you are much more aware of any nibbling you're doing while cooking. I call this nibbling the "hand-to-mouth" diet disease!

People often complain they have difficulty being a guest in someone's home when that someone uses the old "kill the company" manners. You do not have to eat everything you are served. "No" can be a wonderful word when properly used. It is not impolite to ask for your salad without dressing or your vegetables without sauce. If you had a food allergy you would not hesitate to tell your host or hostess about it. Maybe you could say you are allergic to high-calorie foods because they make you break out in fat!

Remember the diet rule: "Stop when you are no longer hungry. Never continue to eat until you are uncomfortably full." If you can only manage a bite or two of your dessert, simply tell your host or hostess that the meal was so delicious that you simply don't have room for more.

DINING OUT

I have to travel a great deal, which forces me to eat breakfast, lunch and dinner far more frequently in restaurants than I eat at home. I would like to share a discovery of mine with you—I have never yet been in a restaurant, of any type, anyplace in the world, where they *made* me finish everything on my plate!

The average restaurant serves portions designed for a man at least six-feet tall and approaching 200 pounds. If you must eat out a large percentage of the time and you are not this tall, then you simply cannot eat everything you are served at every meal or, indeed, you *will* soon approach 200 pounds, regardless of your height.

Keep in mind when you are in a restaurant that you can order exactly what you want. At breakfast, if you prefer one piece of toast instead of two, order only one. If it is difficult for you to stop eating when you are satisfied rather than full, this can be a wonderful way to regulate your appetite. Even if you have to pay for two pieces of toast, consider it money well spent for the privilege of feeling better and more comfortable when you are through with your breakfast. Almost all restaurants offer fresh oranges or grapefruit or some other fresh fruit, whole-wheat toast or cereal and milk or cottage cheese. More and more restaurants have non-fat milk and low-fat cottage cheese available. The secret of eating a healthy breakfast out is daring to be different. Just because everyone is having either bacon and eggs and buttered toast, or just a cup of coffee with a donut or a sweet roll, does not mean that *you* cannot have fresh fruit and cottage cheese. Recently when I was in a hotel coffee shop in the mid-west, I ordered half a grapefruit, whole-wheat toast, dry, and cottage cheese. The waitress told me that they did not have grapefruit or any other fresh fruit but that they did have canned grapefruit juice. She also told me that they did not have cottage cheese for breakfast. I asked her if they served cottage cheese for lunch and she said, "Oh yes, we have a fresh fruit and cottage cheese salad on our luncheon menu." After discussing my dilemma for several minutes, I convinced her that since the fruit and cottage cheese had to be in the kitchen in a refrigerator if they were going to serve it for lunch, perhaps someone could get it out and fix me a fresh fruit and cottage cheese salad for my breakfast. "A salad for breakfast?" I assured her that I frequently had salad for breakfast and that I would still like to order the dry whole-wheat toast, served on the side. If you are ever in this situation and they can't come up with fresh fruit, order an unsweetened juice. Fruit juice is never as nutritious a choice as the whole fruit because it lacks fiber, but when nothing else is available it is certainly an acceptable alternative.

Eating out when you are on the Food Lover's Basic Diet actually may prove a help rather than a hindrance, particularly if you are trying to break the bad habit of nibbling while you cook or of eating leftovers while you're cleaning up. It keeps you out of the kitchen and puts you in control, ordering exactly what you want.

In restaurants, cream soups are almost always made with cream and thus are high in calories, fat and cholesterol. Many soups are oversalted as well and are much too high in sodium. A clear consommé is the rare exception to this rule and even then some restaurants tend to serve them too salty.

When ordering a salad, always order the dressing on the side. If you are eating out while on the Basic Diet, ask for lemon wedges and vinegar. If you eat in the same restaurant every day for lunch, you may want to ask if they will keep a jar of Jones Dressing in their refrigerator for you. You will also be amazed to find how good many salads taste without any dressing at all. Most vinaigrette-type dressings are very high in calories because of the oil; Roquefort and bleu cheese dressings have even more calories and are also very high in sodium. Nothing is worse than getting a soggy, overdressed salad with the lettuce literally swimming in dressing.

When ordering anything on a menu that comes with a sauce, ask for your sauce to be served on the side. The same holds for dressings. This way you control how much sauce or dressing is used rather than leaving it up to someone else's discretion. You will discover that a very little bit of sauce or dressing goes a long way toward enhancing the flavor of a salad or an entrée. Plus, you may occasionally get a sauce you don't like, and you will be spared having it all over your food.

It is generally best to order à la carte in restaurants when possible. This way you can decide what you really want and work the rest of your meal around it. You may prefer to have only a salad and an appetizer. Appetizers are served in small portions and are routinely less expensive than entrées. For variety, you may even want to have two appetizers rather than one entrée.

Remember the concept of conscious eating. Plan exactly what you're going to have before ordering. Always think about what you are going to do after you eat as well. Thinking about how you want to feel at the end of the meal is important in making appropriate menu selections. If you are going back to work, you want to be alert and effective, not lethargic and so sluggish that doing anything will be a great effort. If you are going on to the theater or a ball game, you don't want to feel full or sleepy. If you are going to play golf or tennis, you will want to feel lithe and energetic. So order *and* eat with your future activity in mind (this kind of conscious planning for the future also helps tremendously in other areas of your life!)

When your meal arrives, stick to your plan and consciously enjoy everything you are eating. Balance your own menu. If you really want a heavy entrée like Beef Wellington, then you certainly don't want to order escargots in garlic butter as an appetizer and a salad with bleu cheese dressing; nor do you want to follow it with a rich cheesecake for dessert.

While you are on the Basic Diet, order your fish, meat or poultry baked or broiled without added fat. The same advice goes for vegetables—without butter or sauce. Even in cafeterias you can ask for your food without sauce.

If you must eat out every day and the restaurant where you go does not have any whole-grain bread or baked potatoes, take a roll or some bread with you. This suggestion applies to fresh fruit as well, though you can nearly always order some sort of fresh fruit. Nevertheless, if you know the particular restaurant you're going to does not offer fruit, take some along with you. As I said once before, you may find eating out is a real help until you learn not to be tempted to munch while cooking.

Once you are on the Lifetime Diet, dining out in restaurants becomes a real adventure. You now can order anything you want because you have learned *how*. No temporary lapses of memory are allowed! If you go hog wild—in other words, make a pig of yourself—that's exactly what you will feel like when you leave. Nothing is fun when you are too full! With this in mind, these are your guidelines for eating in restaurants: Think through both the meal and the activity to follow before ordering; avoid combining calorie-laden courses; and order all sauces and salad dressings on the side.

In restaurants specializing in a particular cuisine such as French, Italian or German, where you may not be familiar with all of the dishes on the menu, do not hesitate to ask questions. When eating in Oriental restaurants, always order your meal prepared without MSG (monosodium glutamate).

Do not allow yourself to be intimidated by a waiter or waitress no matter what the restaurant. You are the customer, and you are the one who is ordering the meal, eating the meal *and* paying for the meal. You would not go into a department store and let a salesperson sell you a suit that was too small, or in a color you didn't like, because you feared hurting the person's feelings. So why should you eat a salad with dressing poured over it when you ordered it on the side? Or accept a well-done steak you requested rare? Or keep the broccoli with hollandaise sauce when you asked for it plain, without even any butter? There is certainly a great difference between being assertive enough to be in control of the situation in a restaurant and being rude and obnoxious.

Remember that the "I have to eat all of it because I am paying for it" syndrome relates directly to the "all of the poor starving children in the world" notion I talked about earlier. Members of the Clean Plate Club don't need to carry cards—they are easily recognized because they are all *fat!*

When dining out with a friend who is also on the Food Lover's Diet, the situation is much easier. Since most restaurants serve portions of fish, poultry and meat at least twice as large as you're allowed on the diet, you can order one entrée and ask to split it. Even if they have a service charge for dividing the entrée, it is still less expensive and less wasteful than each of you leaving half your order on your plate.

ECONOMIC ADVANTAGES

A wonderful dividend on the Food Lover's Diet is the money you are going to save. The economic advantages of buying only basic unprocessed products, such as fresh fruits and vegetables, whole-grain bakery goods and cereal, and limiting the amount of animal protein and dairy products in your diet is enormous. If you have been in the habit of buying canned and frozen vegetables, frozen TV dinners and other processed foods that come already prepared, I can promise you that you will be cutting your grocery bill by at least a third when shopping for the Food Lover's Diet. To further cut your food costs, use the shopping tips in the section on entertaining.

Frozen broccoli, for example, is four times more expensive per pound than fresh broccoli in the store where I shop. Frozen peas are five to six times more expensive than fresh peas in the pod. Buying all of the ingredients for the Chow Mein recipe in this book brings the serving cost to one-tenth of what it is if you buy a frozen chow mein dinner, and you get the advantage of all the vitamins and minerals available in the fresh product without any of the added chemical preservatives and high sodium content found in the frozen product. In other words, you pay far less money for far more nutritional value.

You will save enough money on groceries in just two weeks on the Food Lover's Diet to more than pay for the purchase of this book. This in itself is a wonderful reason for going on this diet!

Special Diets

DIABETIC DIET

The Food Lover's Diet is designed perfectly for diabetics on the Diabetes Exchange Diet; however, before going on this or any other diet it is advisable for anyone with diabetes to check with his or her physician to make certain that it is acceptable.

All of the Food Lists at the back of the book are based on the Exchange Diet Program approved by the American Diabetes Association. The Exchange Diet Program is a system of grouping foods according to the amounts of carbohydrates, protein, fat and calories they contain.

Although I use the Exchange Diet for the diet program in the Food Lover's Diet, elsewhere I have made three changes in terminology, which seem to be more easily understood by most people.

First, the term "exchange" is changed to "portion." *Second,* the food groups usually called "bread exchange" is titled "starches," which better describes the entire food group, particularly in a diet program where the importance of the complex carbohydrates, or starches, is stressed. *Third,* the food group usually called "meat exchange" is titled "proteins," again because it better describes the entire category listed as "protein portion."

The diet should be used exactly the same way the Exchange Diet is used. Your doctor tells you how many portions of *each* food group you may have each day. You then may choose from the specific food group the portion you wish for your meals that day. The variety is practically endless! All you have to remember is that you must have the proper number of portions from *each* food group *each* day.

On the Vegetable Portion List, I have based the figures on one cup, unless otherwise specified, rather than one-half cup of every vegetable. The reason for this is that one cup more realistically reflects the number of calories in the serving sizes of most vegetables.

On the Low-Fat Protein Portion List, under Fish and Seafood, I have used amounts over one ounce for many of the low-fat fish and seafood items, again because they more realistically reflect the numbers of calories usually consumed.

EXPLAINING THE EXCHANGE DIET

There are six basic types of food:
- Foods containing only carbohydrates are called Fruit *Exchanges* or Fruit *Portions*.
- Foods containing carbohydrates and small amounts of protein are called Vegetable *Exchanges* or Vegetable *Portions*.
- Foods containing larger amounts of carbohydrates and protein are called Bread *Exchanges* or Starch *Portions*.
- Foods containing nearly equal amounts of carbohydrates and proteins are called Milk *Exchanges* or Milk *Portions*. They are divided into three groups: non-fat, low-fat and whole, depending upon the amount of fat each contains.
- Foods containing protein and some fat are called Meat *Exchanges* or Protein *Portions*. They are also divided into three groups: low-fat, medium-fat and high-fat, depending upon the amount of fat each contains.
- Foods containing mostly fat are called Fat *Exchanges* or Fat *Portions*.

"Exchange" is the term given to a specified amount of a certain type of food. One Exchange may be "exchanged" for any other specified amount within the same group because it has the same food value and the same number of calories. For example: One small orange is listed as one Fruit Exchange; two apricots are also one Fruit Exchange. If you are allowed only one Fruit Exchange for lunch, you may want one small orange or you may want only one-half orange and one apricot, which also equals one Fruit Exchange. It doesn't matter which fruit or fruits you choose so long as the amount you eat adds up to one Fruit Exchange.

The same thing is true of all the Exchange Lists. One Bread Exchange can also be one-half cup rice. If you are allowed only one Bread Exchange for lunch, you may want one slice of bread toasted or you may want one-half cup rice instead. If you want both the toast and rice, you can only have one-half slice toast and one-quarter cup rice, which together equal one Bread Exchange.

As a general rule, trades should not be made between different Exchange groups. However, it is good to know which food groups can be exchanged for other food groups in case of emergencies.

It is easiest to interchange Fruit and Bread Exchanges. Also, it is the most frequently necessary type of sustitution.

1 Fruit Exchange = 2/3 Bread Exchange
1 Bread Exchange = 1-1/2 Fruit Exchanges

For example: If fruit were not available, you could eat two-thirds slice of bread instead of the fruit. Or if you needed another Bread Exchange, you could eat three dates instead of half an English muffin, or one-and-a-half Fruit Exchanges instead of one Bread Exchange!

You can also interchange Bread Exchanges and Vegetable Exchanges:

1 Vegetable Exchange = 1/3 Bread Exchange
1 Bread Exchange = 3 Vegetable Exchanges

For example: You can substitute one soda cracker for one cup cooked broccoli or have three-quarters cup cooked peas instead of one bread slice.

One eight-ounce glass of low-fat milk equals one Low-Fat Milk Exchange and may be substituted for one Bread Exchange plus one Low-Fat Meat Exchange. Or, if you don't have milk, you may have one generous Fruit Exchange plus one Low-Fat Meat Exchange. See why you often hear milk called the complete food!

Remember these interchanges are for emergencies only and should not be used regularly.

At first you may have trouble planning menus in which the exact amounts of everything you are supposed to be eating come out right. The biggest problem is that it is impossible to get away from using fractions, or parts of Exchanges, in recipes. To make this problem as simple as possible, I have simplified the fractions throughout the book.

They are either 1/4, 1/2 or 3/4 of the whole Exchange portion—and in the Milk Exchange category I have added 1/8, as I explain in the introduction to the Calculating Calories Chart. This chart will help you add up the calories for fractions of Exchanges without stopping to do the arithmetic each time.

The following menu planning guide appears in both of my books, *The Calculating Cook* and *More Calculated Cooking*. An easy way to plan your menus is to think of an Exchange like this:

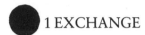 1 EXCHANGE

Then as you use each part of the Exchange, think of it like this:

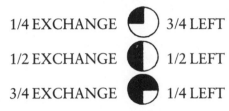

1/4 EXCHANGE   3/4 LEFT

1/2 EXCHANGE   1/2 LEFT

3/4 EXCHANGE   1/4 LEFT

For example, you may have 1/4 of a Bread Exchange in your main dish. So think of it like this:

1/4 EXCHANGE   3/4 LEFT

Go a step further and use another 1/2 Bread Exchange in your salad (croutons).
Now you have:

3/4 EXCHANGE   1/4 LEFT

No need to fret over how to use the remaining 1/4 Bread Exchange in a gourmet fashion. Just eat 2 tablespoons of rice or 1/4 slice of bread and forget it.

If you learn to keep this mental picture, even going through a cafeteria line will cease to be a nightmare. You first pick up a salad with 1/4 cup pineapple and 1/2 cup of low-fat cottage cheese:

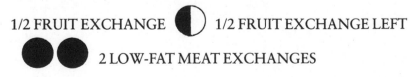

1/2 FRUIT EXCHANGE   1/2 FRUIT EXCHANGE LEFT

2 LOW-FAT MEAT EXCHANGES

Now you don't have any more Meat Exchanges left because you only have 2 for that meal, but you still have:

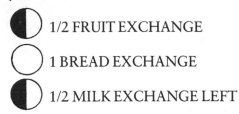

1/2 FRUIT EXCHANGE

1 BREAD EXCHANGE

1/2 MILK EXCHANGE LEFT

Then you see 1/4 cup blueberries. Great, now your Fruit Exchange looks like this. Just as it should!

Take 1/2 pint of milk, pour half of it over your blueberries:

Take 2 graham crackers:

Eat them with your blueberries and milk for dessert: You've had a perfectly balanced lunch.

HYPOGLYCEMIA

People with hypoglycemia follow basically the same Exchange Diet as people with diabetes. The only difference is that they frequently eat smaller, more frequent meals. If you have hypoglycemia and want to go on the Food Lover's Diet, check with your doctor and get his or her approval first.

LOW-CHOLESTEROL DIET

All of the information in the cholesterol section in the chapter on Diet Restrictions is important on a low-cholesterol diet. If you are on a low-cholesterol diet, read that section first and then apply the further restrictions listed in this section.

The American Heart Association suggests limiting cholesterol to 300 milligrams or less per day. If your personal diet prescription is for less than that, the Food Lover's Diet will still be perfectly acceptable for you, with the possible exception of the egg on Sunday. Use one-quarter cup of an egg substitute for that meal instead of the egg. The Food Lover's Diets are all limited to 260 milligrams or less of cholesterol per day.

When you go from the Food Lover's Basic Diet to the Lifetime Diet, pay special attention to the milligrams of cholesterol in planning your own menus. The menu planning charts should be very helpful. Also all recipes in this book give the amounts of cholesterol per serving portion, which will help in your computation. In the Lifetime Diet chapter, you will learn how to calculate the amounts of cholesterol for yourself in your own recipes by using the Food Lists I have provided.

LOW-SODIUM DIET

The sodium discussion in the chapter on Diet Restrictions contains a great deal of valuable information for people on low-sodium diets. If you are on a totally salt-free, very low-sodium diet, please read that material first, and afterwards the additional information in this section which more specifically relates to your special problem.

With the high level of sodium consumption in this country, reducing your sodium intake to very low levels presents a great challenge unless you cook for yourself consistently.

When you are put on a low-sodium diet, head for the nearest health food store and ask to see all of their very low-sodium products. If the selection is small, copy the names and addresses of the manufacturers of those items that are available and write for a complete list of their low-sodium products. The Low Sodium Pantry, 4901 Auburn Avenue, Bethesda, Maryland 20014, will send you a brochure upon request, as will the Chicago Dietetic Supply, P. O. Box 40, La Grange, Illinois 60525. Label reading is especially important for those on low-sodium diets. Watch for ingredients which contain the word "sodium" and avoid those products with such ingredients.

If you don't have a health food store nearby, check the diet foods in your grocery store. More and more low-sodium items are appearing as the public begins to buy such things. I hope this demand will continue to hasten the supply. When I wrote *The Secrets of Salt-Free Cooking*, there were several sources of both liquid and powdered low-sodium milk. The Low Sodium Pantry carries the LSM low-sodium milk in quart cans. The price is high, but demand may eventually help to bring it down.

The Food Lists in the back of the book show the milligrams of sodium per portion, and I am sure your doctor has told you which foods to avoid. On the Food Lover's Diet, your relish tray shouldn't have celery, but you will find many other vegetables on the Vegetable Portion List that are low in sodium. Buy dry-curd cottage cheese if you can, or rinse low-fat cottage cheese in a strainer, sieve or cheesecloth to reduce the sodium content.

Where my recipes call for salt or soy sauce, you will have to improvise with the herbs and spices (see the Spice Chart). I do not use sodium extravagantly in any of my recipes; however, the recipes in my *Secrets of Salt-Free Cooking* were written with sodium restiction as the primary objective.

Learning to cook without salt is probably one of the toughest problems you'll face in the kitchen—in the beginning. But after the first week or two, you'll actually prefer less salt and so will your whole household. Fill the salt shakers with something else of your choosing—or better yet, put them away where they can't be found! Become skillful with herbs and spices and experiment with the lemon juice-pure crystalline fructose combination I dicuss in the section on refined sugar.

Buy an assortment of plastic containers so you can carry your own salad dressings, unsalted margarine, crackers, melba toast, low-sodium whole-wheat bread and other items which experience will teach you are not going to be available *yet* in most of the places where you go to eat out. (I say "yet" because I think the age of enlightenment is about to dawn on the subject of sodium.) A thermos bag can be useful if no refrigerator is available or if your destination is some distance away from home.

Fast-food restaurants aren't equipped to vary their fare, so steer clear of them, as well as some of the ethnic restaurants that specialize in highly seasoned and spiced foods. They would find it almost impossible, without a lot of notice and instruction, to cook without their customary seasonings and oils.

When you are invited to dinner, let your hostess know that you'll want your salad dressing and any sauces on the side and offer to bring your own. If she's really your friend, she'll think this is a good idea. Just present your containers upon arrival and enjoy being a guest.

Ask for low-sodium meals on airplanes when you make your reservations; and when you check in for your flight, find out if your special meal has in fact been boarded.

When making hotel reservations, ask for a room with a refrigerator or ask for permission to store some of your margarine, dressings, bread, etc., in a kitchen refrigerator during your stay. The chef may have a sodium problem too!

You must be firm in your insistence that your food be cooked to your specifications. Call ahead to see if this is possible. If not, go to a restaurant that understands the reason for your request and will cooperate. Insist upon a salad with fresh, uncooked vegetables; find out if the meat, poultry or fish are precooked for last-minute browning or if they are raw and can be cooked to order. Avoid ordering soup or consommé in restaurants. They contain salt and usually in larger amounts than is even necessary for good flavor. Avoid ordering pasta in restaurants because it is cooked in salted water. Many desserts also contain salt; therefore, fresh fruit is always your best choice. Ask to have your vegetables steamed or cooked in unsalted water with no sauce or butter added to them.

Explain to the person taking your order that you are not trying to be difficult or picky—but that you have a serious health problem and would really appreciate his or her cooperation.

If you are on an extremely low-sodium diet, it is a good idea to check with your local water department about the sodium content of your tap. The sodium content of local water supplies varies greatly from one area to another. If there are more than 30 milligrams of sodium per quart, I advise using distilled water for both drinking and cooking. Home water softeners are great for your dishwasher and will keep spots off your water glasses (soft water is even good for washing your dog) but softeners also add a great deal of sodium to the water; therefore, such water should not be used for drinking or cooking. In fact, if you are on a low-sodium diet, you should be drinking distilled water *all* the time.

When ordering bottled water in a restaurant, be sure to choose a natural low-sodium sparkling water. Artificially carbonated water is higher in sodium because sodium is required for the water to retain its carbonation; without sodium soda water loses its bubbles as soon as the bottle is opened.

HERPES SIMPLEX

For many years, people suffering from Herpes Simplex have endured painful, unsightly cold sores, or fever blisters, as they are sometimes called, with only a few over-the-counter remedies, none of which helped much. There has been much publicity recently about Herpes, which has now been divided into two classes, Herpes I, the cold-sore type, and Herpes II, a genital strain of Herpes which is spread much like venereal disease. Today, far more medical attention is being focused on the problem of Herpes and more research is being funded.

One of the major breakthroughs in Herpes is the realization that diet plays an important role in controlling it. We talked already about the nine essential amino acids which the body cannot produce. One of them is lysine. Apparently the keys to the nutritional control of Herpes are two amino acids, lysine and arganine. Although our body cannot produce lysine, arganine is one of the non-essential amino acids which the body can manufacture. The Herpes virus grows well when supplied with arganine. Conversely, lysine inhibits the growth of the Herpes virus. The obvious way to combat Herpes is by increasing our consumption of lysine-high foods and eliminating as much as possible foods high in arganine. High-arganine foods include nuts, seeds and chocolate. High-lysine foods include fresh fish, canned fish, chicken and beef (see the following chart). Lysine can also be purchased in pill form without prescription in most drug stores and health food stores. One 500-milligram capsule per day of lysine may prevent a recurrence of the virus when it is inactive. Some doctors recommend as much as 1500 milligrams of lysine in three doses, 500 milligrams each morning, noon and night, to stop a Herpes attack; others recommend twice that much. When buying lysine, be sure to get the right kind—L-Lysine. If the label reads simply "Lysine" you're probably getting a less potent mixture; D-Lysine is ineffective against Herpes.

The Food Lover's Diet is ideally suited to people wishing to control Herpes Simplex I or II because almost all high-arganine foods are also high in fat content and calories; whereas high-lysine foods are all acceptable on the diet.

Since Herpes is still very much under study, I suggest you check with your doctor before taking lysine as a preventive measure; how-

ever, following the guidelines of the diet is certainly in no way harmful
and will help to keep you slim forever, Herpes or no Herpes!

FOODS TO EAT
  (HIGH IN LYSINE)
Beans, cooked (except garbanzos)
Bean sprouts
  (especially mung beans)
Beef
Brewer's yeast
Chicken
Cottage cheese, dry
Crustaceans
Fish, fresh and canned
  (highest in lysine)
Lamb
Milk
Soybeans

FOODS TO AVOID
  (HIGH IN ARGANINE)
Carob powder
Chocolate
Cocoa
Garbanzo beans
Nuts
Peanut butter
Seeds

Questions and Answers

Q. *Why is this diet safe compared to other diets?*
A. Because it is perfectly balanced, containing foods from all of the food groups, thus ensuring an adequate amount of all the necessary vitamins and minerals as well as an adequate amount of fiber.

Q. *I am a diabetic. Is this diet safe for me?*
A. Yes. This diet is perfectly balanced for a diabetic; however, if you have diabetes you should not go on this or any other diet program without first discussing it with your doctor.

Q. *Is this diet safe for children?*
A. Yes. The Food Lover's Diet is a perfectly balanced diet containing enough of all the necessary food groups for good nutrition for the whole family.

Q. *Will I be weaker and more likely to get sick on this diet?*
A. No. You should feel better, look better and have more energy on this diet than you have ever had before.

Q. *Can I stay on the Basic Diet as long as I want?*
A. Yes. The Basic Diet is a perfectly balanced diet for all your nutritional needs. It is safe to stay on it until you have reached your desired weight.

Q. *How much weight per week will I lose on the diet?*
A. The average weight loss on the Basic Diet is between 10 and 14

pounds over two weeks. This will vary depending on the amounts of the allowed foods you eat and the amount of excercise you get.

Q. *Will exercise help me lose weight or not?*
A. Certainly exercise will help you lose weight, because it will help you to burn up calories faster; however, some people get discouraged when the weight loss shown on the scale is not as dramatic once they start getting a lot of regular exercise. This is because they are losing fat and building muscle at the same time and muscle weighs more than fat.

Q. *Why can you eat all the potatoes, etc., you want? Aren't starchy foods fattening?*
A. The complex carbohydrates, or "starch foods," are actually not as "fattening" as many other foods. Many people have the misconception that potatoes are high in calories, when in fact there are only four calories per gram in potatoes; it is the fats that are added to potatoes (at nine calories per gram) that make them fattening. The average baked potato contains only about 140 calories; however, most people put two or three tablespoons of butter, as well as sour cream and sometimes even chopped bacon on top, which can bring the total calorie count to as high as 600 calories—making the potato fattening indeed.

Q. *If I eat only a limited amount of meat, etc., will I get an adequate amount of protein on this diet?*
A. The Food Lover's Diet is between 20 and 25 percent protein, which is certainly enough for good health.

Q. *You limit meat, fish, etc., on the Food Lover's Diet. I thought protein burned up fat and helped you lose weight. Is this not true?*
A. I limit all animal protein in order to control the amount of saturated fat and cholesterol in the diet. Protein does *not* burn up fat. Taking in fewer calories than you use for energy is the way to get rid of fat.

Q. *Why do you specify non-fat milk on the Food Lover's Diet? Isn't whole milk more nutritious than non-fat milk?*
A. No. Eight ounces of whole milk contain the equivalent of two rounded teaspoons of butterfat. This is 10 grams of fat, or 90 calories. The same eight-ounce glass of milk also contains 12 grams of carbo-

hydrate and eight grams of protein for a total of 170 calories. This means that there are three times as many calories available in fat as there are in protein, and twice as many as in carbohydrates. The butterfat is a saturated fat which is not good for anyone, at any age, and in fact is potentially dangerous to your health. Low-fat milk has the equivalent of one rounded teaspoon of butterfat or five grams of fat, which is 45 calories in fat, while non-fat milk does not have any fat, only carbohydrates and protein.

Q. If I eat more meat than specified on the diet one day, can I make up for it by eating no meat the next day?
A. If you eat more meat on one day than you should, just get back on track and follow the diet as closely as you can on the following days.

Q. Isn't a certain amount of fat (such as safflower oil) necessary for good health?
A. Yes. A certain amount of the polyunsaturated fatty acid, linoleic acid, is necessary; however, there is enough of this fatty acid in the Food Lover's Diet to maintain good health.

Q. I thought a little fat was necessary for a good complexion. Will my skin suffer on this diet?
A. It is not fat that is necessary for a good complexion; it is the moisture in your skin that keeps it clear, young looking and resilient. Drinking eight glasses of water a day will give you a beautiful complexion.

Q. Will losing weight on this diet cause me to look older? I have a friend whose face seemed to sag after she lost weight.
A. Absolutely not. Most people, after losing weight on the Food Lover's Diet and following it exactly, report that their friends think they have had a face lift. Skeptical? Just you wait and see!

Q. Why don't you allow margarine? I thought it was non-fattening.
A. All fats contain nine calories per gram and will make you fat faster than anything else. (See the Fat Portion Lists in the back of the book.) Polyunsaturated margarine has other advantages over butter, but fewer calories is not one of them.

Q. Can I substitute some butter for the cheese or milk on the diet?

A. No. Butter is a saturated fat and cannot be substituted for the protein available in cheese or milk.

Q. Can I skip the milk on the diet?
A. Yes. You can skip the milk on the diet by substituting one-half cup of low-fat cottage cheese, partially skimmed ricotta cheese or hoop cheese for each one cup of your milk allowance.

Q. I'm allergic to fish. What can I substitute for the diet menus that call for fish?
A. Chicken is a wonderful substitute for fish and can be used with great success in all of the fish recipes provided in the Party Diet section.

Q. Do I have to eat everything listed on each menu?
A. Yes. It is important to eat some of each type of food on each menu. You do not have to eat very much of the food, but in order to maintain a well-balanced diet containing all of the necessary vitamins and minerals and fiber it is necessary to eat at least some of everything.

Q. Can I skip breakfast and eat more for lunch or dinner?
A. No. Breakfast is a very important meal and is essential for a nutritionally sound diet.

Q. Can I save some items on the lunch or dinner menu for mid-afternoon or late-night snacks?
A. Yes. You can save the milk allowance to use as a midmorning, midafternoon or late-night snack if you wish. Also, you may eat any of the foods on the Free-Food List (page 53) for snacks whenever you wish.

Q. Can I substitute coffee or tea for some of the daily eight glasses of water required on the diet?
A. No. When you are losing weight your body is throwing off more toxins or impure body waste products than at any other time. In order to keep these toxins or impurities washed out of the system, you must drink lots of water. It also helps your kidneys function more efficiently and will keep your skin clear and looking younger. Coffee and tea are both loaded with impurities of their own and certainly cannot be used to help rid the body of impurities.

Q. Does drinking coffee or tea affect weight loss?
A. The caffeine in coffee and tea has a tendency to lower the blood sugar while stimulating the adrenal gland to produce adrenalin. As soon as the "hype" from the adrenalin has worn off, you are left hungrier than you were before and therefore more apt to eat things you shouldn't between meals.

Q. What's the difference between fructose and regular sugar? In a pinch can I substitute?
A. The difference between fructose and regular sugar (sucrose) is that sucrose contains a higher percentage of glucose. The higher the percentage of glucose in a refined sugar, the more rapid the insulin response will be and therefore the more rapid the drop in blood sugar and the associated feeling of hunger. Therefore, it is best to avoid regular sugar altogether. However, if you do substitute regular sugar for fructose, the general rule is to use one-third more of the sucrose for the same degree of sweetness that you get from fructose.

Q. Does sugar make you gain weight?
A. Sugar causes a rapid rise in blood sugar with a corresponding rapid drop. This makes you feel hungry, and hunger causes most people to eat things they ordinarily would not and should not eat. Also, most sweets, such as ice cream, pies, cakes, cookies, etc., also have a high *fat* content and are therefore very high in calories.

Q. Does restricting salt in the diet help you lose weight?
A. No. Salt is not a food and does not contain calories; however, salt does cause fluid retention, which can make your weight on the scale higher. If you are used to eating a lot of salt and then start eliminating as much salt as possible from your diet, you will probably register less on the scale because you will not be retaining as much fluid. Too much salt can also be dangerous to your health.

Q. I have no self-discipline; are there any foods that help compulsive eaters?
A. Yes. The complex carbohydrates. They are more filling, more satisfying and will keep you from feeling hungry for longer periods of time. The Food Lover's Diet should be perfect for you!

Q. What if I blow it one day—how can I recover my losses?
A. Simply by getting right back on track and following the rules of the diet the following day. Remember the definition of diet is "food and drink habitually taken." That means you're always on a diet, you *can't* go off it. You can just make a mistake.

Q. Do you have any tips for midnight snackers?
A. Yes. Keep bowls of the chopped vegetables on your Free-Food List in the refrigerator so that when you get the "munchies" at midnight you will not end up eating ice cream or that leftover pie.

Q. I have always gained weight rapidly when I have gone off other diets. Will this happen with the Food Lover's Diet?
A. Absolutely not. You will learn on the Food Lover's Diet how to maintain your weight loss even after you start on the Lifetime Diet and you can eat or drink anything you want.

Q. What if my family refuses to eat the foods allowed on the diet? Should I make separate meals?
A. No. It won't be necessary. You can prepare exactly the same foods, leaving the high-fat sauces and salad dressings off your own portion.

PART III

FOOD LOVER'S RECIPES

Here you will find all of the recipes referred to throughout the book. Also, I have included some of my own favorite recipes that can be incorporated into your own menu planning.

STOCKS, SAUCES AND TOPPINGS

BEEF STOCK

3 pounds beef or veal bones
1 pound beef, cut of choice (optional)
2 carrots, scraped and cut into pieces
2 celery stalks, without leaves
1 onion, cut in half
1 tomato, cut in half
3 garlic gloves
2 parsley sprigs
2 whole cloves
1/4 teaspoon dried thyme, crushed, using a mortar and pestle
1/4 teaspoon dried marjoram, crushed, using a mortar and pestle
1 bay leaf
10 peppercorns
1 teaspoon salt
Defatted Beef Drippings, page 123 (optional)

Put the bones and enough cold water to cover by 1 inch in a large soup kettle. Bring to a boil. Simmer slowly for 5 minutes, then remove and discard any scum that has formed on the surface. Add the meat, vegetables and spices and enough additional cold water to cover by 1 inch. Cover, leaving the lid ajar about 1 inch to allow the steam to escape. Simmer very slowly for at least 5 hours (10 hours is even better). When the stock is finished cooking, strain it and allow it to come to room temperature.

Refrigerate, uncovered, overnight. The next morning remove and discard the fat that has hardened on the surface. After removing every bit of fat, warm the stock until it becomes liquid. Strain the liquid and add salt to taste. If the flavor is too weak, boil to evaporate more of the water and concentrate its strength, or add defatted drippings.

Store the stock in the freezer, putting some of it in ice cube trays for individual servings (2 cubes equal 1/4 cup). The stock may also be stored in a tightly covered container in the refrigerator for not more than 2 days.

MAKES about 2-1/2 quarts (10 cups). 1 cup contains approximately:
Tr. cholesterol when defatted/ 200 mg. sodium.
Calories negligible

CHICKEN STOCK: Substitute 3 pounds of chicken parts (wings, backs, etc.), for the beef or veal bones and 1 whole stewing chicken (optional) for the pound of meat. Omit the tomato, thyme and marjoram and the defatted beef drippings. Proceed according to the recipe.
LOW SODIUM: Omit the salt and use distilled water. Increase the thyme and marjoram to 1 teaspoon each and add 1 teaspoon celery seeds. This reduces the sodium to a negligible factor.

BROWN SAUCE

2 cups beef stock
1-1/2 teaspoons finely chopped shallots
1/4 cup burgundy
2 tablespoons sherry
2 tablespoons dry white wine (I prefer chablis)
2 tablespoons cornstarch
2 tablespoons cold water
1/4 teaspoon salt
Dash of freshly ground black pepper
1 teaspoon Kitchen Bouquet

In a saucepan, heat the beef stock. In another pan combine the chopped shallots and wines and heat over fairly high heat, boiling it until it has reduced by one-third in volume. When reduced, add the heated beef stock to the wine and then lower the heat to medium. Allow the mixture to come again to a simmering boil. Mix the cornstarch and water until completely dissolved. Add the cornstarch mixture to the sauce, mixing thoroughly using a wire whisk. Season to taste with salt and pepper. To get the rich dark brown color associated with the classic French brown sauce, add the Kitchen Bouquet.

MAKES 2 scant cups. 1/2 cup contains approximately:
1/4 starch portion/ 18 calories/ 0 cholesterol/ 286 mg. sodium

NOTE: Brown Sauce is an essential ingredient for such classics as Coq au Vin, Osso Buco and Cassoulet. It can also make a simple broiled ground-round patty an epicurean delight.

DEFATTED DRIPPINGS

If you love gravy, but don't eat it because it's *fat, fat, fat,* then one of your problems is solved. Simply defat your drippings.

All drippings are defatted in the same manner. After cooking your roast beef, leg of lamb, chicken, turkey or whatever, remove it from the roasting pan and pour the drippings into a bowl. Put the bowl in the refrigerator until the drippings are cold and all of the fat has solidified on the top. Remove the fat and you have defatted drippings.

If you are in a hurry to serve your roast beef au jus, just put the drippings in the freezer instead of the refrigerator (put the roast in the oven to keep it warm). After about 20 minutes you can remove the fat, heat the jus and serve. Freeze any defatted drippings you are not using for the meal. They can be added to stocks for extra flavor and are good for making low-calorie gravies.

NOTE: Defatted Drippings, even though visible fat is removed, contain a trace of cholesterol, and the sodium content will depend upon the seasoning you have used on your meat, in addition to the sodium content of the meat itself.

SKINNY GRAVY
(BEEF, CHICKEN, TURKEY)

1 cup Defatted Drippings, page 123,
or 1 cup concentrated Beef, Chicken or Turkey Stock
1 tablespoon cornstarch or arrowroot
2 tablespoons minced onion, browned, or
1 tablespoon dehydrated onion flakes (optional)

Heat the defatted drippings in a saucepan. As soon as they become liquid, put a little of the liquid in a cup and stir in the cornstarch to form a smooth paste. Pour the cornstarch mixture into the saucepan, blending well. Add the browned onion, if desired, and simmer until the gravy thickens slightly, stirring occasionally.

NOTE: Beef or Chicken or Turkey Stock, page 121, can be stored in ice cube trays in the freezer and used for individual servings of this gravy. For a 1/4 cup serving use 2 stock "ice cubes," 1/4 teaspoon cornstarch or arrowroot and 1 teaspoon minced onion, browned, or 1/2 teaspoon dehydrated onion flakes (optional).

MAKES approximately 1 cup. 1/4 cup contains approximately:
0 cholesterol/ 21 mg. sodium/ Calories negligible

VEGETABLE STOCK

2 stalks celery with leaves, chopped
2 leeks, thinly sliced
4 carrots, chopped
2 onions, thinly sliced
2 cabbage leaves, shredded
1 head lettuce, cored and shredded
4 sprigs parsley with stems, chopped
1 teaspoon salt
1 teaspoon dried thyme
1 bay leaf
8 cups water

Combine all ingredients in a large kettle and slowly bring to a boil. Skim and cover, leaving the lid ajar, and simmer for about 1 hour. Strain into a bowl, allowing the stock to drain freely. Save the vegetables to use as a side dish or purée them for dips.

MAKES 1-1/2 quarts. 1 cup contains approximately:
0 cholesterol/ 300 mg. sodium
Calories negligible

COCONUT SAUCE

1 envelope (1 tablespoon) unflavored gelatin
2 tablespoons cold water
1/4 cup boiling water
2 cups non-fat milk
1 teaspoon vanilla extract
1 teaspoon coconut extract

Soften the gelatin in the cold water. Add the boiling water and stir until the gelatin is completely dissolved. Add the milk and mix well. Place the gelatin-milk mixture in a covered container in the refrigerator. When it is thickened it is ready to use. Place the gelatin-milk mixture in a blender container. Add the vanilla extract and coconut extract and blend until smooth. Allow to stand a few minutes to thicken before serving.

MAKES 2 cups. 1/4 cup contains approximately:
1/4 non-fat milk portion/ 20 calories
2 mg. cholesterol/ 31 mg. sodium

DILL SAUCE

1 cup plain non-fat yogurt
1 teaspoon dried tarragon, crushed, using a mortar and pestle
1 tablespoon dried dill weed, crushed, using a mortar and pestle
1/4 teaspoon salt

Combine all ingredients in a bowl and mix thoroughly. Store, covered, in the refrigerator. This sauce is best prepared the day before you plan to use it.

MAKES 1 cup. 1/4 cup contains approximately:
1/4 non-fat milk portion/ 20 calories
4 mg. cholesterol/ 29 mg. sodium

MARINARA SAUCE

1 29-ounce can tomato sauce
2 cups water
1 large onion, finely chopped
2 cloves garlic, finely minced
3/4 teaspoon dried oregano, crushed, using a mortar and pestle
3/4 teaspoon dried basil, crushed, using a mortar and pestle
Dash cayenne pepper

Combine all ingredients in a saucepan and bring to a boil. Reduce the heat and simmer, uncovered, for a least 2 hours.

MAKES about 6 cups. 1/2 cup contains approximately:
1 vegetable portion/ 25 calories/ 0 cholesterol
840 mg. sodium with regular tomato sauce
(50 mg. sodium with unsalted tomato sauce)

SAUTERNE SAUCE

1/2 cup Mock Sour Cream, page 133
1/2 cup plain non-fat yogurt
2 tablespoons sauterne

Mix together and refrigerate all day or overnight before serving.

MAKES 1 cup sauce. 1/4 cup contains approximately:
1/2 low-fat protein portion/ 1/8 non-fat milk portion
38 calories/ 3 mg. cholesterol/ 136 mg. sodium

BASIC WHITE SAUCE

2 cups non-fat milk
1 tablespoon corn oil margarine
2-1/2 tablespoons sifted all-purpose flour
1/8 teaspoon salt

Put the milk in a saucepan on low heat and bring to the boiling point. In another saucepan, melt the margarine and add the flour, stirring constantly. Cook, stirring, for 3 minutes. *Do not brown.* Remove the flour-margarine mixture from the heat and add all the simmering milk, stirring constantly with a wire whisk. Put the sauce back on low heat and cook slowly for 15 minutes, stirring occasionally. If you wish a thicker sauce, cook it a little longer. Add salt and mix thoroughly. If there are lumps in the sauce (though there shouldn't be by this method), whirl in blender container until smooth.

MAKES 1-1/2 cups. 3/4 cup contains approximately:
1-1/2 fat portions/ 1/2 starch portion/ 1 non-fat milk portion
183 calories/ 5 mg. cholesterol/ 603 mg. sodium

FAT-FREE WHITE SAUCE

1-1/2 cups non-fat milk
1/4 teaspoon salt
Dash white pepper (optional)
3 tablespoons cream of rice

Combine the milk, salt and white pepper in a saucepan and bring just to the boiling point. Add the cream of rice and stir for 30 seconds. Remove from the heat, cover and allow to stand for 5 minutes. Using a wire whisk, beat until smooth. Season as you would any white sauce and use immediately as a sauce or for other recipes. Store, covered, in the refrigerator and reheat as needed.

MAKES 1-1/2 cups sauce. 1/4 cup contains approximately:
1/4 starch portion/ 1/4 non-fat portion
38 calories/ 2 mg. cholesterol
114 mg. sodium

CURRIED YOGURT DRESSING

1 cup plain non-fat yogurt
1/2 teaspoon curry powder
1/4 teaspoon salt
1 teaspoon pure crystalline fructose

Put all ingredients in a mixing bowl and mix thoroughly. Refrigerate.

MAKES 1 cup. 1/4 cup contains approximately:
1/4 non-fat milk portion/ 20 calories
4 mg. cholesterol/ 20 mg. sodium

CURRIED COCONUT YOGURT DRESSING: Add 1/4 teaspoon coconut extract.
CURRIED GINGER YOGURT DRESSING: Add 1/8 teaspoon ground ginger.

JONES BASIC DRESSING

1/4 teaspoon salt
1/4 cup red wine vinegar
1 teaspoon pure crystalline fructose
1/8 teaspoon freshly ground black pepper
1/4 teaspoon garlic powder
1 teaspoon Worcestershire sauce
2 teaspoons Dijon-style mustard
2 teaspoons fresh lemon juice
1/2 cup water

Dissolve the salt in the vinegar, then add all of the remaining ingredients and mix well. Pour into a jar with a tightly fitting lid and shake vigorously for 1 full minute. Store in the refrigerator.

MAKES 1 scant cup. 2 tablespoons contain approximately:
0 cholesterol/ 82 mg. sodium/ Calories negligible

JONES TARRAGON DRESSING: Add 1 teaspoon dried tarragon, crushed, using a mortar and pestle.

JONES CUMIN DRESSING: Add 1/4 teaspoon ground cumin to the Basic Dressing.

JONES ITALIAN DRESSING: Add 3/4 teaspoon dried oregano, 1/2 teaspoon dried basil and 1/2 teaspoon dried tarragon, crushed, using a mortar and pestle.

JONES CURRY DRESSING: Add 1/2 teaspoon curry powder to the Basic Dressing.

LIFETIME DIET VARIATION: Add 2 tablespoons corn oil.

2 tablespoons contain approximately:
3/4 fat portion/ 34 calories/ 0 cholesterol/ 82 mg. sodium

LOW-SODIUM VARIATION: Omit the salt. Add 2 more teaspoons of fresh lemon juice.

2 tablespoons contain approximately:
0 cholesterol/21 mg. sodium
Calories negligible.

To further reduce the sodium, you can omit the Dijon-style mustard and add 1/4 teaspoon dry mustard.

2 tablespoons contain approximately:
0 cholesterol/ 4 mg. sodium/ Calories negligible.

JONES PINEAPPLE–GINGER DRESSING

1 cup unsweetened pineapple juice
1/4 cup water
2 tablespoons rice vinegar
1 tablespoon reduced sodium soy sauce or tamari
1 teaspoon garlic powder
1 tablespoon finely chopped fresh ginger root or
1/2 teaspoon ground ginger

Combine all ingredients in a jar with a tight-fitting lid. Mix thoroughly and store in the refrigerator for at least 12 hours before using.

MAKES 1-1/2 cups. 2 tablespoons contain approximately:
1/4 fruit portion/ 10 calories/ 0 cholesterol/ 51 mg. sodium

VARIATION: If using cider vinegar, use only 1 tablespoon instead of 2.

JONES TOMATO DRESSING

1 16-ounce can tomatoes, undrained (2 cups)
2 tablespoons fresh lemon juice
2 tablespoons red wine vinegar
1 teaspoon dried oregano, crushed, using a mortar and pestle
1/2 teaspoon dried basil, crushed, using a mortar and pestle
1/2 teaspoon dried tarragon, crushed, using a mortar and pestle
1/2 teaspoon pure crystalline fructose
1/4 teaspoon garlic powder
1/4 teaspoon onion powder
1/4 teaspoon salt
1/4 teaspoon freshly ground black pepper

Put all ingredients in a blender container and blend until smooth. Store in the refrigerator in a covered container.

MAKES 2-1/2 cups. 2 tablespoons contain approximately:
1/4 vegetable portion/ 7 calories
0 cholesterol/ 54 mg. sodium

LOW-SODIUM VARIATION: Use unsalted canned tomatoes. Increase to 2-1/2 tablespoons lemon juice and increase to 1 teaspoon pure crystalline fructose; omit salt. 2 tablespoons will contain 4 mg. of sodium. Everything else will remain the same.

LOW-CALORIE CATSUP

4 cups tomato juice
1/4 cup wine vinegar
2 whole garlic cloves
3/4 teaspoon pure crystalline fructose

Put the tomato juice, vinegar and garlic in a saucepan and bring to a boil. Reduce heat to very low and simmer for about 3-1/2 hours, or until sauce reaches desired thickness. Remove from heat and cool to room temperature. Remove garlic cloves and add the fructose. Store in a glass or plastic container in the refrigerator.

Making your own catsup saves calories. One-half cup of tomato juice is only 1 vegetable portion. Two tablespoons of commercial catsup equal 1 fruit portion; 3 tablespoons equal 1 starch portion. When you reduce 4 cups of tomato juice to 1-1/2 cups as you do in this recipe, you get 2 tablespoons catsup for only 1/4 vegetable portion and 7 calories.

MAKES 1-1/2 cups. 2 tablespoons contain approximately:
1/4 vegetable portion/ 7 calories/ 0 cholesterol/ 81 mg. sodium

MAJOR JONES CHUTNEY

5 cups peeled and diced cooking apples (6 apples or 2 pounds)
1 medium onion, peeled and diced
1/2 cup raisins
1/2 cup chopped dried figs (about 5)
2 cups cider vinegar
1 cup pure crystalline fructose
2 teaspoons salt
1 tablespoon ground ginger
1/2 teaspoon cayenne pepper
2 tablespoons pickling spices tied in a cheesecloth bag
(discarded after cooking)

Combine all ingredients in a large saucepan and bring to a boil. Reduce heat and simmer uncovered for 2 hours. Refrigerate.

MAKES 4 cups. 1 tablespoon contains approximately:
1/2 fruit portion/ 20 calories/ 0 cholesterol/ 62 mg. sodium

MUSTARD DIP

1/2 cup plain non-fat yogurt
1 tablespoon prepared spicy brown mustard
1 teaspoon pure crystalline fructose
1/2 teaspoon cider vinegar
1/8 teaspoon garlic powder

Place all ingredients in a bowl and mix thoroughly. This dip is excellent for raw or cooked vegetables. It is also a good sauce for hot vegetables, baked potatoes, fish, poultry and meat.

> MAKES 1/2 cup dip. 1/4 cup contains approximately:
> 1/4 non-fat milk portion/ 20 calories
> Tr. cholesterol/ 153 mg. sodium

VARIATION: For a milder dip, use 1/2 teaspoon rice vinegar instead of cider vinegar.

TOFU DRESSING OR DIP

> 8 ounces tofu
> 1 8-ounce can crushed pineapple packed in natural juice
> 3/4 teaspoon dried basil, crushed, using a mortar and pestle
> 3/4 teaspoon dried marjoram, crushed, using a mortar and pestle
> 1/8 teaspoon ground white pepper
> 2 teaspoons soy sauce

Combine all ingredients in a blender container and blend until smooth. Refrigerate for several hours before using if possible, as the flavor will improve.

This is a delicious salad dressing, particularly on fruit salad. It is also excellent served with cottage cheese, ricotta or hoop cheese. Serve it as a dip for raw vegetables or a sauce on cooked vegetables, fish or poultry.

> MAKES 2 cups. 1/4 cup contains approximately:
> 1/4 medium-fat protein portion/ 1/4 fruit portion
> 29 calories/ 0 cholesterol/ 87 mg. sodium

BREAKFAST CHEESE

> 1-1/2 cups partially skimmed ricotta cheese
> 1/4 cup plain non-fat yogurt

Combine all ingredients in a blender container or a food processor with a metal blade and blend until completely smooth. Refrigerate, covered, for 1 day before using.

MAKES 1-1/2 cups. 1/4 cup contains approximately:
1 low-fat protein portion/ 55 calories
18 mg. cholesterol/ 51 mg. sodium

VARIATION: Substitute low-fat cottage cheese or hoop cheese for the partially skimmed ricotta cheese. I personally do not think the cottage cheese or hoop cheese Breakfast Cheese is as good as the ricotta version.

JELLED MILK

1 envelope (1 tablespoon) unflavored gelatin
2 tablespoons cold water
1/4 cup boiling water
1 cup non-fat milk

Soften the gelatin in the cold water. Add the boiling water and stir until the gelatin is completely dissolved. Add the milk and mix well. Place the gelatin-milk mixture in a covered container in the refrigerator. When it is jelled, mixture is ready to use.

Blend Jelled Milk with an equal amount of non-fat milk in the blender and use over fruit or cereal. The thick, creamy consistency will make the milk seem richer.

MAKES 1 cup. 1 cup contains approximately:
1 non-fat milk portion/ 80 calories
5 mg. cholesterol/ 127 mg. sodium

MOCK SOUR CREAM

1 cup low-fat cottage cheese
2 tablespoons buttermilk
2 teaspoons fresh lemon juice

Put all ingredients in a blender container or a food processor with a metal blade and blend until completely smooth. Even when you think it's smooth enough, blend a little longer for a better result.

MAKES 1 cup. 1/4 cup contains approximately:
1 low-fat protein portion/ 55 calories
3 mg. cholesterol/ 243 mg. sodium

JONES DIPS

Adding the following to 1 cup Mock Sour Cream:
CURRY DIP: Add 1/2 teaspoon curry powder and 1/8 teaspoon ground ginger to the Mock Sour Cream.
MEXICAN DIP: Add 1/2 teaspoon chili powder, 1/4 teaspoon ground cumin, 1/4 teaspoon garlic powder and a dash of Tabasco (optional).
TARRAGON DIP: Add 3/4 teaspoon dried tarragon, crushed, using a mortar and pestle.
DILL DIP: Add 1/4 teaspoon dried tarragon and 1/2 teaspoon dried dill weed, crushed, using a mortar and pestle.
ONION DIP: Add 3/4 teaspoon onion powder and 1 teaspoon instant dried minced onion and a dash of Tabasco (optional).

LIFETIME DIET DIP VARIATIONS:
DESSERT DIP: Substitute 2 tablespoons non-fat milk for the buttermilk in the basic Mock Sour Cream recipe. Add 2 tablespoons pure crystalline fructose, 1-1/2 teaspoons vanilla extract and 1/2 teaspoon ground cinnamon (optional). This dip is wonderful with fresh fruit for dessert or spread on French toast and pancakes.
1/4 cup contains approximately:
1 low-fat protein portion/ 1/2 fruit portion/ 75 calories
3 mg. cholesterol/ 238 mg. sodium
MOCK MAYONNAISE: Add 2 tablespoons corn oil, 1 tablespoon red wine vinegar and 1/2 teaspoon dry mustard to the Mock Sour Cream.
1/4 cup contains approximately:
1 low-fat protein portion/ 1-1/2 fat portions
83 calories/ 3 mg. cholesterol/ 244 mg. sodium

NON-FAT YOGURT

2 cups instant non-fat dry milk
4 quarts non-fat milk
1 cup plain low-fat yogurt

Combine the dry and liquid non-fat milk in a large saucepan and mix thoroughly. Heat slowly for 15 minutes over medium heat. *Do not boil*. Remove from the heat and allow to cool for 25 minutes. Skim off the film that forms on the surface. Add the yogurt and mix well into the milk mixture.

Sterilize a large container (or containers) in boiling water. Pour the mixture into a sterilized container for 3 to 6 hours. If you have a gas stove, place the container in the oven and the pilot light will keep it at the proper temperature. If you do not have a gas stove, place the container in warm water that you replace or replenish regularly to maintain the temperature.

When the mixture has thickened enough to hold together (test by tilting the container slightly), refrigerate for 4 or 5 hours to thicken to the proper yogurt consistency.

This homemade yogurt can be used in any recipe calling for yogurt. If it makes more yogurt than you can use in a week's time, reduce the recipe accordingly.

MAKES 4 quarts yogurt. 1 cup contains approximately:
1 non-fat milk portion/ 80 calories
5 mg. cholesterol/ 127 mg. sodium

WHIPPED "CREAM"

2/3 cup canned, skimmed evaporated milk
2 teaspoons unflavored gelatin
2 tablespoons cold water
1/4 cup boiling water

Pour the milk into a bowl and place in the freezer for about 30 minutes. Soften the gelatin in the cold water in a saucepan for 5 minutes. Add the boiling water and stir until the gelatin is completely dissolved; set aside. Beat the chilled milk until very thick. Gradually add the gelatin mixture and beat until the mixture forms soft peaks. Serve immediately. (This can only be refrigerated for 1 hour before losing its whipped consistency.)

MAKES 4 cups. 1/2 cup contains approximately:
1/4 non-fat milk portion/ 20 calories
Tr. cholesterol/ 28 mg. sodium

SOUPS

BLUEBERRY SOUP

3 cups fresh or unsweetened frozen blueberries
1 8-ounce can unsweetened crushed pineapple, undrained
1 teaspoon fresh lemon juice
1/2 teaspoon vanilla extract
8 teaspoons plain non-fat yogurt
Fresh mint sprigs for garnish

Put 2 cups of blueberries in a blender container. Set the remaining cup of blueberries aside to add later. Add all other ingredients to the blueberries in the blender container, except the yogurt and mint sprigs, and blend until smooth.

Add the remaining cup of blueberries to the soup in the blender and mix well with a spoon or rubber spatula. *Do not blend.* Pour the soup into chilled bowls and put 1 teaspoon of non-fat yogurt on top of each serving. Garnish each serving with a sprig of fresh mint.

MAKES 8 servings. Each serving contains approximately:
1 fruit portion/ 40 calories/ 1 mg. cholesterol/ 2 mg. sodium

EGG FLOWER SOUP

3 cups chicken stock
2 egg whites
2 tablespoons chopped chives or green onion tops

Bring the chicken stock to a boil. Beat the egg whites until they are frothy. Slowly pour the beaten egg whites into the boiling chicken stock. Stir constantly with a fork or wire whisk. Continue to stir the soup rapidly until the egg whites are shredded and look like long strings. Serve very hot in heated bowls. Sprinkle the top of each bowl of soup with chopped chives or green onion tops. (You may add a little salt-reduced soy sauce if desired; this will increase the sodium level.)

MAKES 4 servings. Each serving contains approximately:
Tr. cholesterol/ 173 mg. sodium/ Calories negligible

GAZPACHO

2 cups tomato juice
1/4 onion, minced
1/2 small green bell pepper, minced
1/4 large cucumber, peeled and diced
1 canned green chili, seeds removed and chopped
3/4 teaspoon Worcestershire sauce
1/2 garlic clove, minced
1/4 teaspoon seasoned salt
1 drop Tabasco (optional)
1/8 teaspoon freshly ground black pepper
1 small tomato, finely diced
1 tablespoon chopped chives or green onion tops
1 lemon cut in wedges

Put 1 cup of tomato juice and all other ingredients except the diced tomato, chives and lemon wedges in the blender container. Blend well. Slowly add the remaining cup of tomato juice to the blender. Pour the mixture into a bowl and add the diced tomato. Garnish with the chopped chives and serve with the lemon wedges.

MAKES 4 servings. Each serving contains approximately:
1 vegetable portion/ 25 calories/ 0 cholesterol/ 392 mg. sodium

VARIATION: For a more chunky texture, combine all ingredients in a mixing bowl and mix thoroughly instead of blending. This chunky textured version makes an excellent salsa dressing for salads, fish, meat or poultry.

SHERRIED CONSOMMÉ

2 egg whites
4 cups chicken stock
1 bay leaf
1 tablespoon chopped fresh parsley
1 tablespoon sherry

Beat the egg whites with a wire whisk until they are slightly foamy. Add 1 cup of the cold stock to the egg whites and beat lightly together. Put the rest of the stock in a pan with all other ingredients except the sherry. Bring to a boil and remove from the heat. Slowly pour the egg white-stock mixture into the stock, stirring with a wire whisk. Put the pan back on very low heat and mix gently until it starts to simmer. Simmer slowly for 40 minutes. Line a strainer with 2 or 3 layers of damp cheesecloth. Ladle the consommé through the cheesecloth. Allow it to drain undisturbed until it has all seeped through. Before serving, add the sherry and mix thoroughly.

MAKES 4 servings (1 cup each). Each serving contains approximately:
1/2 low-fat protein portion/ 28 calories
2 mg. cholesterol/ 224 mg. sodium

STRACCIATELLE ALLA ROMANA

4 cups chicken stock
2 egg whites
1/8 teaspoon ground nutmeg
1 tablespoon grated Romano cheese
2 tablespoons minced fresh parsley

Bring the chicken stock to a boil in a saucepan. Combine the egg whites, nutmeg and Romano cheese and beat thoroughly. Add the parsley to the beaten egg mixture and pour the entire mixture into the boiling stock, stirring continuously until the eggs are cooked. (This only takes a minute.) Immediately ladle the soup into 6 bowls and serve.

MAKES 6 servings. Each serving contains approximately:
1/2 low-fat protein portion/ 28 calories
2 mg. cholesterol/ 160 mg. sodium

VEGETABLES AND VEGETARIAN ENTRÉES

DIRECTIONS FOR STEAMING VEGETABLES

When steaming vegetables, always make certain that the steamer basket is above the level of the water and that the water is boiling rapidly before the vegetables are covered and timing is begun.

Once the vegetables have steamed for the correct length of time, immediately place them under cold running water. This stops the cooking quickly and preserves color and texture.

Whether you are going to be serving vegetables hot or cold, they can be prepared in advance and stored, covered, in the refrigerator. Many of the recipes in this book call for steamed vegetables, and by preparing them in advance, preparation at meal time can be greatly shortened. When reheating steamed vegetables, be careful not to overcook them in the reheating process or they will lose both their crispness and their color.

In the following steaming chart, the time indicated for steaming each vegetable will produce a crisp-tender result. Mushy, colorless vegetables are not only tasteless, they have been robbed of much of their nutritional value by overcooking.

FRESH VEGETABLE STEAMING CHART

VEGETABLE	MINUTES	VEGETABLE	MINUTES
Asparagus	5	Leeks	5
Beans:		Lettuce	1–2
green	5	Lotus root	
lima	5	1/4-inch slices	25
string or snap	5	Mushrooms	2
Bean sprouts	1–2	Mustard, fresh	1–2
Beet greens	3–5	Okra	5
Beets, quartered	15	Onions:	
Black radish,		green tops	3
1/2-inch slices	5	whole	5
Breadfruit	10	Palm hearts	5
Broccoli:		Parsley	1–2
flowerets	3–5	Pea pods	3
branches	5	Peas	3–5
Brussels sprouts	5	Peppers:	
Cabbage, quartered	5	chili	2–3
Carrots, 1/2-inch slices	5	green and red bell	2
Cauliflower:		Pimientos	2
flowerets	3	Poke	3
whole	5	Potatoes:	
Celery root	3–4	sweet, 1/2-inch slices	15
Celery stalks	10	white, 1/2-inch slices	10
Chard	1–2	Pumpkin, cut up	5
Chayote	3	Radishes	5
Chicory	1–2	Rhubarb	5
Chives	2–3	Romaine lettuce	1–2
Collards	1–2	Rutabagas	8
Corn	3	Shallots	2
Coriander (cilantro)	1–2	Spinach	1–2
Cucumber	2–3	Squash:	
Eggplant, cut up	5	acorn or Hubbard, cut up	5
Garlic	5	summer or zucchini	3
Jerusalem artichokes	8	Tomatoes	3
Jicama	10	Turnips, quartered	8
Kale	1–2	Water chestnuts	8
Kohlrabi, quartered	8–10	Watercress	1–2

SPROUTING

It should come as no surprise that all seeds can be sprouted. Most sprouts are excellent snack foods. They are rich in vitamins, and I recommend that you have a bag of them in your refrigerator at all times to munch on along with your free vegetables.

The most common sprouts in grocery and health food stores are alfalfa and bean sprouts; however there are a number of others— sunflower seeds, triticale, mung beans, lentils, Chinese cabbage, wheat berries, etc.—that are also very good and easy to grow and harvest. Your health food store will have a variety of seeds for sprouting and also paraphernalia used for cultivating them; but a plain glass jar with cheesecloth over the top will be good enough for starting out.

Soak the seeds overnight in the glass jar. Then drain off the water and rinse the seeds thoroughly and drain again. Secure the cheesecloth to the top of the jar and place the jar on its side, out of the direct sunlight. Rinse the seeds a couple of times a day, and again return the jar to its side, out of the light. You can start nibbling after two days in most cases.

When making large amounts of sprouts, enough for a loaf of Sprouted Wheat Berry Bread for example, I use a large cookie sheet with sides and place a damp cheesecloth on it. Then I spread the seeds, which have been soaked overnight and drained, over the damp cheese- cloth and cover with another piece of damp cheesecloth. In the morn- ing and evening, I sprinkle enough water over the cheesecloth to keep it moist, and in three days I have eight cups of wheat berry sprouts from one cup of wheat berries. The sprouts grow down through the cheesecloth and you have to pull them out; the whole process makes quite a heavy "blanket" of sprouts. According to my favorite health food store, sprouting wheat berries increases their Vitamin C content by 600 percent.

The quality of seeds varies, so yields will also vary. Alfalfa is the most expansive (one-quarter cup of seeds gives you four cups of sprouts in two days). Sunflower seeds only produce about three-quarters cup from one-quarter cup of seeds in the same length of time, but if allowed to continue growing will do better in three or four days. Experiment.

After the sprouting is well underway (two to four days) place the sprouts in the refrigerator and use for snacks as well as for ingredients in salads, sandwiches and other dishes. They have a very low calorie density and a very high nutritional density.

Black-eyed pea sprouts taste like fresh peas and are good in salads. Mung beans are especially popular and practically start sprouting during the soaking process. Try a variety.

YIELDS PER 1/4 CUP SEEDS IN TWO DAYS

Alfalfa: 8 cups
Black radish: 5 cups
Buckwheat: 1-3/4 cups
Chinese cabbage: 3 cups
Fenugreek: 6 cups
Lentils: 3 cups

Mung beans: 3-1/2 cups
Pinto beans: 1-1/4 cups
Sunflower seeds: 1-3/4 cups
Triticale: 1-1/4 cups
Wheat berries: 4 cups
Whole peas: 2 cups

ASPARAGUS VINAIGRETTE

20 fresh asparagus spears
1/2 cup Jones Tarragon Dressing, page 128
1 2-ounce jar pimientos
2 tablespoons capers

Wash the asparagus thoroughly and break off the tough end sections. Steam the spears for about 3 minutes, or until crisp-tender but not limp. Cool to room temperature and place in a glass baking dish, all spears pointing in the same direction (this makes removal for serving much simpler). Pour the Jones Tarragon Dressing over the asparagus and cover tightly with foil.

Refrigerate all day or overnight to thoroughly marinate the asparagus. To serve, place on chilled asparagus dishes or salad plates and place the pimiento strips and capers equally over each serving.

MAKES 4 servings. Each serving contains approximately:
1/2 vegetable portion/ 13 calories/ 0 cholesterol/ 1 mg. sodium

HERBED VEGETABLE MEDLEY

2 cups assorted steamed vegetables
(any combination or a single vegetable)
3 tablespoons chicken stock
1/8 teaspoon salt
1/2 teaspoon dried basil, crushed, using a mortar and pestle
2 tablespoons finely chopped fresh parsley
2 tablespoons finely chopped chives or green onion tops

Steam the vegetables until just crisp-tender. Time will vary from one vegetable to another. See Steaming Chart. This recipe is also an excellent way to use leftover steamed vegetables. Heat the chicken stock in a skillet. Add the salt, basil, parsley and chives or green onion tops and mix thoroughly. Add the cooked vegetables and mix thoroughly. Heat just to serving temperature. Overheating will destroy both the color and texture of the vegetables.

MAKES 4 servings. Each serving contains approximately:
1/2 vegetable portion/ 13 calories
0 cholesterol/ 80 mg. sodium

NOTE: Use this recipe to prepare Herbed Carrots and Herbed Zucchini and Onions.

TOMATO PROVENÇAL

2 large tomatoes
1/4 cup buttermilk
2 teaspoons grated Romano or Parmesan cheese
Salt
Freshly ground black pepper

Cut the tomatoes into halves and remove the seeds. (If very large tomatoes cut in 1/2-inch slices.) Drip 1 tablespoon of buttermilk onto each tomato half. Sprinkle the top of each with Romano or Parmesan cheese, salt and freshly ground black pepper. Put the tomatoes in a

400° oven for 15 minutes. Then broil until lightly browned. This dish is also good served cold; and it is wonderful for lunch.

MAKES 4 servings. Each serving contains approximately:
1 vegetable portion/ 25 calories
Tr. cholesterol/ 104 mg. sodium

VARIATIONS: Add a dash of dried oregano, basil, tarragon, garlic or rosemary if you wish.

CURRIED TOFU AND PINEAPPLE SALAD

1 16-ounce can pineapple chunks packed in natural juice
1 pound tofu cut in 1/2-inch cubes
5 cups torn Boston lettuce
1 cup Curried Yogurt Dressing, page 128
Lettuce leaves for bowl liners

Pour the pineapple and all the juice from the can into a large bowl. Add the tofu. Cover and refrigerate for several hours before serving. Drain the pineapple juice from the tofu and pineapple mixture. Combine the pineapple chunks and tofu with the torn lettuce and Curried Yogurt Dressing and toss thoroughly. Serve in cold bowls or on cold plates lined with lettuce leaves.

MAKES 4 servings. Each serving contains approximately:
1 fruit portion/ 1 medium-fat protein portion
1/4 non-fat milk portion/ 135 calories
4 mg. cholesterol/ 41 mg. sodium

CRÊPES FLORENTINE

2 cups partially skimmed ricotta cheese
4 cups chopped cooked spinach (about 4 pounds raw)
1/2 cup finely chopped green onion tops
1/2 teaspoon garlic powder

1/4 teaspoon salt
1 tablespoon grated Romano cheese
8 Blender Crêpes (recipe follows)

Preheat the oven to 350°. Combine all of the ingredients except the Romano cheese and crêpes in a large mixing bowl and blend well. Spoon an equal amount of the mixture evenly down the center of each crêpe and fold both sides of the crêpe over toward the center. Place the crêpes, seam side down, in a glass baking dish. Sprinkle the Romano cheese evenly on top of the crêpes. Bake in a preheated 350° oven for 20 minutes or until the cheese is lightly browned.

MAKES 8 filled crêpes. Each crêpe contains approximately:
1/2 starch portion/ 1 low-fat protein portion
1/2 vegetable portion/ 61 mg. cholesterol/ 137 mg. sodium

BROCCOLI CRÊPES: Substitute 4 cups chopped cooked broccoli for the spinach.

BLENDER CRÊPES

1 cup non-fat milk
3/4 cup whole-wheat flour, sifted
1/4 teaspoon salt
2 eggs, lightly beaten, or 1/2 cup liquid egg substitute
1 teaspoon corn oil margarine

Combine all ingredients, except margarine, in a blender container and blend thoroughly. Melt the margarine in an omelet or crêpe pan over medium heat. Tilt the pan to make sure the entire inner surface is coated. Pour the melted margarine into the blender container with the crêpe batter and mix well.

Pour just enough crêpe batter into the pan to cover the bottom of the pan (about 2 tablespoons) and tilt the pan from side to side to spread the batter evenly. Cook over medium heat until the edges start to curl, then carefully turn the crêpe with a spatula and brown the second side. Repeat until all of the batter is used. To keep the crêpes pliable, put them in a covered casserole in a warm oven.

To freeze the crêpes, put a piece of aluminum foil or waxed paper between each 2 crêpes and wrap them well so that they are not exposed to the air. Before using, bring to room temperature and put them in a preheated 300° oven for 20 minutes, or until they are soft and pliable. If you do not reheat the crêpes, they will break when you try to fold them.

MAKES 12 crêpes (it is not practical to make fewer).
Each crêpe contains approximately:
1/2 starch portion/ 35 calories
42 mg. cholesterol/ 64 mg. sodium

EAST INDIAN CARROT CASSEROLE

1/4 cup Vegetable Stock, page 124
1/4 teaspoon salt
1/2 teaspoon pure crystalline fructose
1 teaspoon curry powder
1 tablespoon freshly grated ginger root or
1/2 teaspoon ground ginger
6 medium-size carrots, grated (3 cups grated carrots)
1/4 cup finely chopped chives or green onion tops
1/2 cup raisins
3 cups low-fat cottage cheese

Heat the Vegetable Stock in a skillet. Add the salt, fructose, curry powder and grated ginger and mix thoroughly. Add the grated carrots, chopped chives and raisins and cook, stirring constantly, until crisp-tender, about 10 minutes. Add the cottage cheese, mix thoroughly and heat just to serving temperature. *Do not bring to a boil!*

MAKES 6 servings. Each serving contains approximately:
2 low-fat protein portions/ 1 vegetable portion/ 3/4 fruit portion
165 calories/ 5 mg. cholesterol/ 610 mg. sodium

HUEVOS RANCHEROS

1/4 cup chicken or vegetable stock
1 onion, chopped
1 green bell pepper, chopped, seeds removed
2 cloves garlic, pressed
1 28-ounce can (3-1/2 cups) peeled tomatoes, chopped,
with the juice from the can
3 green chilies, chopped, with veins and seeds removed
1 teaspoon chili powder
1/2 teaspoon salt
1/3 teaspoon freshly ground black pepper
1 teaspoon dried oregano, crushed, using a mortar and pestle
1/2 teaspoon ground cumin
6 eggs at room temperature
1-1/2 cups (6 ounces) grated Monterey Jack cheese
6 corn tortillas, heated

In a skillet, heat the stock. Add the onion, green pepper and garlic. Cook until the onion is transparent, about 10 minutes. Add all other ingredients except the eggs, cheese and tortillas and cook for 20 minutes.

Carefully break the eggs on top of the sauce, making a little depression for each egg. Sprinkle the grated cheese over the top. Cover and cook for 10 to 12 minutes or until the egg whites are "set" and the cheese is melted. Serve each egg on top of a hot tortilla. Spoon the remaining sauce over the top of each serving.

MAKES 6 servings. Each serving contains approximately:
1 high-fat protein portion/ 1 medium-fat protein portion
1 starch portion/ 1/2 vegetable portion/ 252 calories
277 mg. cholesterol/ 652 mg. sodium

STUFFED TOMATO BOWLS

1/2 cup brown rice
1/4 cup lentils
3/4 cup Vegetable Stock, page 124
1/8 teaspoon salt
1/4 teaspoon dried thyme, crushed, using a mortar and pestle
4 large tomatoes
1/3 cup water chestnuts (1/2 of an 8-ounce can), diced
2 tablespoons finely chopped fresh parsley
3 garlic cloves, minced
1 onion, finely chopped
1 stalk celery, without leaves, finely chopped
1 carrot, finely chopped
1 cup finely chopped mushrooms

Combine the brown rice, lentils, 1/2 cup of Vegetable Stock, salt and thyme and cook until the rice and lentils are done, about 45 minutes. Add a little Vegetable Stock if necessary. Cut the tops from the tomatoes and hollow them out, leaving about 1/4 inch of tomato. Chop the pulp and set aside. Heat the remaining 1/4 cup of Vegetable Stock. Add the water chestnuts, parsley, minced garlic cloves and all the vegetables and the chopped tomato pulp and cook until the vegetables are tender. Combine all the ingredients except the tomato bowls and mix well. Stuff the vegetable/grain mixture (1/2 cup per tomato) into the tomato bowls and place in a baking dish. Bake uncovered for 30 minutes at 350°.

MAKES 4 servings. Each serving contains approximately:
1-3/4 starch portions/ 2-1/2 vegetable portions
186 calories/ 0 cholesterol/ 174 mg. sodium

LENTILS AU GRATIN

1-1/3 cups dried lentils (4 cups cooked)
1 onion, finely chopped
2 cloves garlic, minced
2 cups grated carrots

2 cups drained canned tomatoes
1/2 small bell pepper, seeded and chopped
1 teaspoon salt
1/2 teaspoon freshly ground black pepper
1/4 teaspoon dried marjoram, crushed, using a mortar and pestle
1/4 teaspoon dried thyme, crushed, using a mortar and pestle
3/4 cup (3 ounces) grated Monterey Jack cheese

Place the lentils in water and cook approximately 1 hour or until tender. Preheat the oven to 375°. Place the lentils in a 2-quart casserole. Cook the onion and garlic until soft (about 5 minutes) in a skillet. Add the onion and garlic and all other ingredients except the cheese to the lentils in the casserole. Stir to combine thoroughly and bake, covered, for 1 hour. Uncover the baked casserole and sprinkle the cheese over the top. Return to the oven and bake until the cheese is melted and slightly browned.

MAKES 6 (1-cup) servings. Each serving contains approximately:
1-1/2 starch portions/ 1-1/2 vegetable portions
1/2 high-fat protein portion/ 191 calories
9 mg. cholesterol/ 189 mg. sodium

PALAK PANEER
(EAST INDIAN SPINACH AND CHEESE)

2 pounds spinach, finely chopped, or
4 10-ounce packages frozen chopped spinach
2 teaspoons corn oil
1 teaspoon chili powder
2 teaspoons ground coriander
1 teaspoon ground turmeric
1/2 teaspoon ground ginger
3/4 teaspoon ground cumin
1/2 teaspoon salt
Dash freshly ground black pepper
1 pound farmers' cheese, cut into 1/2-inch cubes

Cook the spinach in a small amount of water until just tender. Drain, reserving the liquid. Put the drained cooked spinach in a blender container and add as much of the cooking liquid as necessary to purée the spinach. Set aside. Heat the oil in a large saucepan. Add all of the remaining ingredients, except the spinach and cheese, and mix thoroughly. Add the puréed spinach to the saucepan and blend well. Add the farmers' cheese and heat just to serving temperature. Be careful not to overheat or the cheese will melt.

   I like this dish served with cold sliced tomatoes, which is the way it was served to me in New Delhi, India, when I was there for the Ninth International Diabetes Federation Congress in 1976.

MAKES 8 servings. Each serving contains approximately:
1/2 vegetable portion/ 1/4 fat portion/ 2 low-fat protein portions
135 calories/ 6 mg. cholesterol
584 mg. sodium with salted cheese
(290 mg. sodium with unsalted cheese)

MOUSSAKA (LIFETIME)

1 large eggplant
Salt
1/4 cup Vegetable Stock, page 124
1 onion, minced
1 garlic clove, finely chopped
2 cups shredded raw zucchini (2 zucchini)
2 tablespoons finely chopped parsley
1/2 cup tomato sauce
1/4 cup dry red wine
1/8 teaspoon ground mace
1/2 teaspoon dried oregano, crushed, using a mortar and pestle
1/4 cup (1 ounce) Monterey Jack cheese, grated
1/4 cup (1 ounce) Parmesan cheese, grated
1-1/2 cups Basic White Sauce, page 126
Parsley sprigs or radish roses for garnish (optional)

Peel the eggplant and cut it lengthwise into 1/2-inch slices. Place in a baking dish and sprinkle both sides with salt. Set aside for at least 1 hour. Heat the Vegetable Stock in a large skillet. Add the onion and garlic and cook until tender. Add the zucchini, parsley, tomato sauce, wine, mace and oregano. Mix thoroughly and simmer for 15 minutes, stirring occasionally. Pour off all of the liquid from the eggplant and steam until it is just fork-tender—about 3 minutes.

To assemble the Moussaka, place one-half of the cooked eggplant over the bottom of a non-stick baking dish. Spread the zucchini mixture evenly over the top of the eggplant. Sprinkle one-half of the Jack cheese and half of the Parmesan cheese over the top. Pour the White Sauce evenly over the top of the eggplant and sprinkle both of the remaining cheeses evenly over the top of the entire dish. Bake, uncovered, in a 350° oven for 45 minutes. Cut into 4 servings. Garnish with parsley sprigs and radish roses on each dish.

MAKES 4 servings. Each serving contains approximately:
2-3/4 vegetable portions/ 1 fat portion
1/2 non-fat milk portion/ 1/4 starch portion
1/4 medium-fat protein portion/ 1/4 high-fat protein portion
215 calories/ 10 mg. cholesterol
872 mg. sodium (675 mg. sodium with unsalted tomato sauce)

VARIATION: For Basic Diet, use Fat-Free White Sauce, page 127. Omit the fat portion and subtract 45 calories per serving.

TOFU STUFFED SPUD

2 baked Idaho potatoes
1 cup tofu (1/2 pound)
1 egg, lightly beaten
1 teaspoon seasoned salt
1/2 cup chopped green onion
1/2 cup sour cream
1/2 cup (2 ounces) grated cheddar cheese

Cut a thin slice from the top of each potato. Remove the pulp from the potatoes, being careful not to tear the shells. Add the tofu to the potato pulp and mash together until thoroughly mixed. Keep the shells warm. Combine the beaten egg and seasoned salt and add to the potato-tofu mixture and mix well. Add all other ingredients and mix well. Heap into the warm potato shells and bake at 350° for 45 minutes.

MAKES 2 servings. Each serving contains approximately:
2 fat portions/ 1-1/2 medium-fat protein portions
1 high-fat protein portion/ 1 starch portion
1/2 vegetable portion/ 371 calories/ 187 mg. cholesterol
1224 mg. sodium

TAMALE PIE

1 onion, finely chopped
1 clove garlic, finely chopped
1 small green chili pepper, seeded and finely chopped
1 16-ounce can tomatoes, chopped, plus all the juice from the can
1-1/4 cups corn kernels
1 tablespoon chili powder
1/4 teaspoon salt
1/4 teaspoon dried oregano, crushed, using a mortar and pestle
1/4 teaspoon dried basil, crushed, using a mortar and pestle
1/4 teaspoon dried thyme, crushed, using a mortar and pestle
1-1/2 cups non-fat milk
1/2 cup yellow cornmeal
1 egg, well beaten
3/4 cup (3 ounces) grated sharp cheddar cheese

Preheat the oven to 350°. Sauté the onions, garlic and green chili pepper in a non-stick pan over very low heat until soft. Add the tomatoes, corn and seasonings and simmer slowly for 10 minutes. Bring the milk to a slow boil. Add the cornmeal and simmer, stirring constantly, until thickened. Add the beaten egg and mix thoroughly. Combine the cornmeal mixture with the vegetable mixture and mix well. Pour into a flat baking dish and bake in a 350° oven for 1 hour. Remove from the oven and sprinkle the grated cheese evenly over the top. Bake for 10 more minutes.

MAKES 4 servings (4-1/2 cups). Each serving contains approximately:
1-3/4 vegetable portions/ 1/2 non-fat milk portion

1-1/2 starch portions/ 3/4 high-fat protein portion
1/4 medium-fat protein portion/ 280 calories
86 mg. cholesterol/ 389 mg. sodium

VEGETARIAN LASAGNA

2 large onions, chopped
1 clove garlic, minced or pressed
1 28-ounce can solid pack tomatoes, drained
2 6-ounce cans Italian tomato paste
1/2 cup chopped fresh parsley
1/2 teaspoon salt
1/4 teaspoon freshly ground black pepper
1 teaspoon dried oregano, crushed, using a mortar and pestle
1/4 teaspoon dried thyme, crushed, using a mortar and pestle
1/4 teaspoon dried marjoram, crushed, using a mortar and pestle
1/4 pound lasagna noodles
1/2 pound ricotta cheese, crumbled
1/4 pound mozzarella cheese, grated
2 tablespoons grated Parmesan cheese

Sauté the onions and garlic in a non-stick pan until tender and slightly brown. Add the tomatoes, tomato paste, parsley, salt, pepper, oregano, thyme and marjoram and simmer for 1 hour, stirring occasionally. While the sauce is simmering, cook the lasagna in 3 quarts of boiling salted water for about 12 minutes. Drain and rinse with cold water in a colander.

Cover the bottom of a baking dish with 1/4 inch of the sauce. Add a layer of lasagna, trimming edges to fit the dish. On top of this, put a layer of ricotta cheese, then a layer of mozzarella cheese and finally sprinkle with Parmesan cheese. Repeat layers until the baking dish is filled. The top layer should be sauce sprinkled with Parmesan cheese. Bake at 350° for 45 minutes.

MAKES 8 servings. Each serving contains approximately:
1 starch portion/ 2-1/2 vegetable portions
1 low-fat protein portion/ 1/2 medium-fat protein portion
226 calories/ 28 mg. cholesterol/ 582 mg. sodium

VEGETARIAN QUICHE

1/4 cup Vegetable Stock, page 124
1 large onion, finely chopped
3 cups coarsely chopped (1/2 pound) broccoli flowerets
2 cups grated (1/2 pound) Monterey Jack or cheddar cheese
3 eggs, lightly beaten
1-1/2 cups low-fat milk

Preheat the oven to 350°. Heat the Vegetable Stock in a large skillet. Add the onion and cook until soft. Add the broccoli and cook for 2 to 3 minutes. Remove from the heat. Spread half the grated cheese evenly over the bottom of a 9-inch pie pan or quiche dish. Spoon the vegetable mixture on top of the cheese. Spread the remaining 1 cup of cheese evenly over the top of the vegetables. Combine the beaten eggs and milk and mix thoroughly. Pour the egg-milk mixture over the top of the quiche. (Low-fat milk is used because quiche has too watery a consistency when made with non-fat milk.) Place the pie pan or quiche dish on a cookie sheet in the center of the preheated oven (quiche often bubbles over during cooking; by placing it on a cookie sheet you will not have to clean the bottom of your oven after baking!). Bake for approximately 1 hour or until golden brown on top. Remove the quiche from the oven and cool for at least 10 minutes before slicing and serving.

MAKES 8 servings. Each serving contains approximately:
1/2 vegetable portion/ 1 high-fat protein portion
1/2 medium-fat protein portion/ 1/4 low-fat milk portion
178 calories/ 115 mg. cholesterol/ 274 mg. sodium

VARIATION: Instead of broccoli, you may prefer to use chopped zucchini, spinach, cauliflower or a combination of vegetables—use your imagination!

VEGETARIAN WHITE CHILI

1/2 pound large dry white beans (1 cup)
4 cups Vegetable Stock, page 124
1 onion, chopped
2 garlic cloves, chopped
1 2-ounce can whole green chili peppers, seeded and chopped
1 teaspoon ground cumin
3/4 teaspoon dried oregano, crushed, using a mortar and pestle
1/2 teaspoon ground coriander
1/4 teaspoon salt
1/8 teaspoon cayenne pepper
2 cups cauliflowerets

Combine the beans, Vegetable Stock, half the onions and the garlic in a large kettle and bring to a boil. Reduce the heat, cover and simmer for 2 hours or until the beans are very tender, adding more Vegetable Stock as needed. Add all other ingredients except the cauliflowerets and cook an additional ten minutes. Add the cauliflowerets and cook until crisp-tender, about 5 minutes. White Chili is delicious and fun to serve because everyone expects chili to be red—not white!

MAKES 4 generous 1-cup servings.
Each serving contains approximately:
1 starch portion/ 1-1/2 vegetable portions
108 calories/ 0 cholesterol/ 437 mg. sodium

VARIATION: Substitute 1-1/2 cups of chopped cooked chicken or turkey for the cauliflower.
Each serving contains approximately:
1 starch portion/ 1 vegetable portion
1-1/2 low-fat protein portions/ 178 calories
34 mg. cholesterol/ 459 mg. sodium

FISH, POULTRY AND MEAT

BAKED TUNA IN TOMATO BOWLS

6 large tomatoes
2 tablespoons chicken stock
1/2 cup finely chopped onion
1/4 cup finely chopped celery
1/2 teaspoon salt
1/4 teaspoon freshly ground black pepper
1 teaspoon dried basil, crushed, using a mortar and pestle
2 7-ounce cans water-packed tuna, drained and flaked
1 tablespoon grated Parmesan cheese

Preheat oven to 375°. Cut a 1/2-inch slice from the stem end of each tomato. Scoop out the pulp and discard the seeds. Chop the pulp and set it aside. Turn the tomato bowls upside down to drain.

Heat the chicken stock in a skillet. Add the onion and celery and sauté until tender. Chop the reserved tomato pulp and add to the skillet. Cook for a few more minutes. Remove from the heat and add the salt, pepper and basil. Then add the tuna and mix well.

Fill each tomato bowl with an equal amount of tuna mixture. Sprinkle a little of the Parmesan cheese over each tomato bowl and arrange the bowls in a baking dish. Bake in the preheated oven for 20 to 25 minutes or until the tomatoes are tender.

MAKES 6 servings. Each serving contains approximately:
1-1/2 vegetable portions/ 3/4 low-fat protein portion
80 calories/ 18 mg. cholesterol/ 192 mg. sodium

BOUILLABAISSE

2 pounds fresh white fish (more than one kind of fish, if possible—
bass, snapper, halibut, turbot, etc.)
2 lemons
Salt
1/4 cup chicken stock

2 large onions, thinly sliced
1 leek, white part only, chopped
2 garlic cloves, minced
3 large tomatoes, peeled, seeded and diced
2 tablespoons chopped parsley
1 stalk celery, finely chopped
1 bay leaf
1/4 teaspoon salt
1/8 teaspoon dried fennel
1/8 teaspoon dried thyme
1/8 teaspoon saffron
Dash freshly ground black pepper
4 cups fish stock or chicken stock
2 cups dry white wine (I like chablis)
8 slices whole-grain French bread

Wash the fish in cold water and pat dry. Place fish in a glass baking dish and squeeze juice of 2 lemons on the fish. Salt lightly on both sides. Cover the dish tightly with aluminum foil or a lid and place in the refrigerator until you plan to cook it.

In a deep kettle or Dutch oven, heat the chicken stock. Add the onions and leeks and cook for 5 minutes. Add the garlic, tomatoes, parsley, celery, bay leaf, salt, fennel, thyme, saffron and pepper. Mix thoroughly and cook for 5 more minutes. Then arrange the fish on top of the vegetables. Pour the stock and dry white wine over the fish. Cover and bring to a boil. Cook for about 8 to 10 minutes, or until the fish has turned white.

The classic way to serve bouillabaisse is to remove the fish from the broth and arrange it on a serving platter. Each guest is then served a bowl of the broth poured over a slice of whole-grain French bread. The fish is passed around and each person helps himself to the fish, putting it in his bowl of broth. You can also divide the fish equally into 8 bowls; then spoon the broth over each serving and pass the bread. The fish remains hot when served this way.

MAKES 8 servings. Each serving contains approximately:
3 low-fat protein portions/ 1 fat portion
1/2 vegetable portion/ 1 starch portion/ 293 calories
54 mg. cholesterol/ 431 mg. sodium

CURRIED SEAFOOD SALAD

4 small heads Boston lettuce
2 apples, diced
2 cups (1 pound) cooked chopped crab, shrimp
or water-packed tuna (or a combination)
1/4 cup raisins
1/2 cup Curried Yogurt Dressing, page 128

Remove the hearts from the heads of lettuce, being careful not to separate or tear the outer leaves. Wash the hearts, tear them into bite-size pieces (approximately 5 cups torn lettuce) and put into a large bowl. Retain the outer leaves for lettuce "bowls" in which to serve the salad. Wash them carefully and place on paper towels in the refrigerator until needed. Add the diced apples to the torn lettuce and mix well. Add the chopped seafood and again mix well. Add the raisins and dressing and toss well. Place each lettuce bowl on a large chilled plate. Divide the salad evenly into the four "bowls."

MAKES 4 servings. Each serving contains approximately:
1 fruit portion/ 2 low-fat protein portions
1/8 non-fat milk portion/ 160 calories
86 mg. cholesterol/ 208 mg. sodium

CURRIED SHRIMP OR CRAB IN PAPAYA CUPS

2 ripe papayas
2 cups flaked cooked crab meat (1 pound) or shrimp (about 2/3 pound)
2 tablespoons finely chopped chives or green onion tops
1/2 teaspoon curry powder
Parsley sprigs for garnish

Cut the papayas in half lengthwise and carefully remove all seeds. Using a melon baller, remove the papaya pulp from the peel, being careful not to tear the peeling. Combine the papaya balls and all other ingredients, except the parsley sprigs, in a mixing bowl and mix well. Divide the mixture equally into the 4 papaya halves. Garnish each papaya cup with a sprig of fresh parsley.

MAKES 4 servings. Each serving contains approximately:
2 low-fat protein portions/ 1-1/2 fruit portions
170 calories/ 96 mg. cholesterol/ 126 mg. sodium

VARIATION: In place of papaya, use 2 small cantaloupes.

POACHED BASS IN DILL SAUCE

2 pounds fresh bass or other firm, white-fleshed fish
1/2 cup finely chopped celery
1/2 cup finely chopped onion
1/2 cup coarsely chopped fresh parsley
1/2 cup dry white wine (preferably chablis)
1/2 cup chicken stock
1/4 teaspoon salt
Dash white pepper
1 cup Dill Sauce, page 125
Fresh dill or parsley sprigs for garnish

Put fish in a large saucepan. Add the celery, onion and parsley. Combine the white wine, chicken stock, salt and white pepper and mix thoroughly. Pour the wine-stock mixture over the fish and vegetables in the saucepan. If the wine-stock mixture does not completely cover the fish, add a little more wine. Slowly bring to a boil. Reduce the heat, cover and cook approximately 8 minutes, or until the flesh of the fish becomes opaque. Remove from heat and allow to cool to room temperature. Remove the fish from the poaching liquid and place in a shallow glass baking dish.

Strain the vegetables from the poaching liquid and add them to the Dill Sauce. Spoon the Dill Sauce-vegetable mixture evenly over the top of the poached fish. To serve, divide and place on individual plates and garnish with fresh dill, if available, or parsley sprigs. This is also good served cold.

MAKES 8 servings. Each serving contains approximately:
2 low-fat protein portions/ 1/4 non-fat milk portion
130 calories/ 58 mg. cholesterol/ 137 mg. sodium

SEAFOOD CHOW MEIN

2 tablespoons salt-reduced soy sauce
4 teaspoons cornstarch
2 tablespoons rice vinegar
1 cup cold water
2 teaspoons pure crystalline fructose
1/4 cup chicken stock
1/2 cup (1/2 8-ounce can) sliced bamboo shoots
2/3 cup (1 8-ounce can) sliced water chestnuts
1 stalk celery without leaves, sliced diagonally
2 cups thinly sliced bok choy (Chinese cabbage), 3 large leaves
2 onions, thinly sliced
1 cup (1/4 pound) sliced fresh mushrooms
1/2 green bell pepper, seeded and thinly sliced
1 cup pea pods
1 pound cooked seafood (shrimp, crab, lobster or a combination)
4 cups bean sprouts
Toasted Chow Mein Noodles (full recipe—page 172)
Chopped chives for garnish (optional)

Put the soy sauce, cornstarch and vinegar in a saucepan and stir until smooth. Slowly stir in the water. Cook over low heat, stirring constantly, until thickened. Add the fructose and set aside.

Heat the chicken stock in a large skillet or a wok. Add all of the vegetables, except the bean sprouts, and the seafood and stir fry for 2 minutes. Cover and cook for another minute. Add the bean sprouts and continue cooking, covered, for approximately 1 more minute. Add the sauce and mix thoroughly. Serve on Toasted Chow Mein Noodles. Garnish each serving with finely chopped chives if desired.

MAKES 4 servings (2 cups each). Each serving contains approximately:
1-1/4 starch portions/ 3 vegetable portions
2-3/4 low-fat protein portions/ 1/4 fruit portion
324 calories/ 113 mg. cholesterol/ 604 mg. sodium

TOFU VEGETARIAN CHOW MEIN: Substitute 1/4 cup Vegetable Stock, page 124, for the chicken stock. Substitute 1 pound of tofu, cut in 3/4-inch cubes, for the 1 pound of seafood.

Each serving contains approximately:
1-1/4 starch portions/ 3 vegetable portions
1 medium-fat protein portion/ 1/4 fruit portion/ 248 calories
0 cholesterol/ 370 mg. sodium

NOTE: I like to marinate the cubed tofu in Vegetable Stock for several hours before using it; it gives it a better flavor.

SHRIMP CURRY WITH CHUTNEY

1 tablespoon corn oil margarine
3 onions, minced
5 tablespoons flour
1 tablespoon curry powder
1 teaspoon salt
1/4 teaspoon ground ginger
1 cup chicken stock
3 cups non-fat milk, warmed
4 cups cooked shrimp (about 1-1/3 pounds)
1/2 cup Major Jones Chutney, page 131

Melt the margarine in a large pot. Add the minced onion and cook until the onion is clear and tender. Combine the flour, curry powder, salt and ground ginger. Add the flour mixture to the onions, stirring constantly, until it becomes a thick paste. Add the chicken stock and stir again until it again becomes a thick paste. Slowly add the warm milk, stirring constantly. Cook slowly, stirring regularly, until the sauce has thickened, about 45 minutes. (It never gets very thick.) Add the shrimp and heat thoroughly. Serve 1 tablespoon of Major Jones Chutney with each serving.

MAKES 8 servings. Each serving contains approximately:
1-3/4 low-fat protein portions/ 1/2 fruit portion
1/2 non-fat milk portion/ 1/2 vegetable portion
1/2 fat portion/ 1/4 starch portion/ 211 calories
85 mg. cholesterol/ 499 mg. sodium

CASHEW CHICKEN SALAD

4 cups chopped cooked chicken
2 cups Jones Pineapple-Ginger Dressing with fresh ginger, page 129
8 cups torn Boston lettuce
2 cups pineapple chunks packed in natural juice, drained
Lettuce leaves for bowl liners
1 cup chopped dry roasted cashew nuts

Marinate the chopped chicken in the Pineapple-Ginger Dressing for at least four hours. Combine the chicken and dressing with the lettuce and pineapple and mix thoroughly. Serve in bowls lined with lettuce leaves and sprinkle 2 tablespoons chopped cashew nuts over top of each serving.

MAKES 8 servings. Each serving contains approximately:
2 low-fat protein portions/ 1-1/2 fruit portions/ 1 fat portion
215 calories/ 52 mg. cholesterol/ 46 mg. sodium

COQ AU VIN

12 small boiling onions, peeled
12 large fresh mushrooms
1/2 cup chicken stock
1 garlic clove, minced
3 whole cooked chicken breasts, halved and skinned
(cooked at 350° for 45 minutes)
2 cups Brown Sauce, page 122

Put the onions in a large saucepan with lightly salted water and cook, covered, for 12 minutes or until fork-tender. Carefully wash the mushrooms and remove the stems. Combine the chicken stock and garlic in a skillet and bring to a boil. Add the mushrooms, reduce the heat and simmer until the mushrooms are tender. Put the cooked chicken and mushrooms in a flat baking dish. Drain the onions and add them to the chicken. Pour the Brown Sauce over the entire dish. Place, uncovered, in a 350° oven for 30 minutes. This dish can be made in the morning and refrigerated until ready for cooking. (I think the flavor is even better when it is made several hours ahead of time.)

MAKES 6 servings. Each serving contains approximately:
1-1/4 vegetable portions/ 1 low-fat protein portion
87 calories/ 23 mg. cholesterol/ 201 mg. sodium

VARIATION: Instead of chicken breasts you may use 6 3-ounce pieces of cooked white turkey meat.

FETTUCCINE CACCIATORE

SAUCE
1 29-ounce can tomato juice
2 cups water
1 large onion, finely chopped
2 cloves garlic, finely chopped
3/4 teaspoon dried oregano, crushed, using a mortar and pestle
3/4 teaspoon dried basil, crushed, using a mortar and pestle
Dash cayenne pepper

2 cups chopped cooked chicken
4 cups (6 ounces) cooked whole-wheat fettuccine noodles

Combine all sauce ingredients in a saucepan and bring to a boil. Reduce the heat and simmer, uncovered, for at least 2 hours. During the last 15 minutes of simmering, add the chopped cooked chicken and mix thoroughly.

Place 1 cup of the cooked whole-wheat fettuccine noodles on each serving plate and divide the chicken-sauce mixture over the top.

MAKES 4 servings. Each serving contains approximately:
2-1/4 vegetable portions/ 2 low-fat protein portions
2 starch portions/ 307 calories/ 45 mg. cholesterol
474 mg. sodium (92 mg. with unsalted juice)

VEGETARIAN FETTUCCINE CACCIATORE: Omit the chicken in the sauce. Add 1-3/4 cups of partially skimmed ricotta cheese to the fettuccine noodles and mix well. Spoon the sauce over each serving. Sprinkle 1 tablespoon of Parmesan cheese over each serving.

Each serving contains approximately:
2-1/4 vegetable portions/ 1-3/4 low-fat protein portions
1/4 medium-fat protein portion/ 2 starch portions/ 313 calories
36 mg. cholesterol/ 478 mg. sodium (96 mg. with unsalted juice)

LEMON CHICKEN IN ENVELOPES

2 whole chicken breasts
Salt
1 teaspoon minced fresh tarragon, or
1/2 teaspoon dried tarragon, crushed, using a mortar and pestle
2 lemons, cut in half
2 cups steamed broccoli or any fresh, green vegetable steamed
(see Steaming Chart, page 140)

Bone, skin and halve the chicken breasts. Remove all visible fat. Place each halved breast on a 12-inch-square piece of aluminum foil and lightly salt both sides of the chicken. Sprinkle each breast evenly with 1/4 teaspoon tarragon. Fold up the aluminum foil, leaving the breast in the center. Then fold each end over twice (about 1 inch for each fold), so that it is possible to squeeze the lemon juice on the chicken without its running out of the foil envelope. Into each envelope squeeze juice of half a lemon. Holding the envelope upright, fold the top side of the envelope over twice, pressing to seal after each fold.

Place all 4 envelopes in a flat baking dish and bake in a 400° oven for approximately 20 minutes. Remove the dish from the oven. Unfold the tops of the envelopes and pour the excess juice over the steamed vegetables. Broccoli just happens to be my favorite vegetable with this sauce, but you may use any green vegetable. Remove the chicken from the envelope and place beside the vegetable on a serving platter or on individual plates and serve immediately. This dish is also good served cold; it is wonderful for a picnic or a brown bag lunch.

MAKES 4 servings. Each serving contains approximately:
1 vegetable portion/ 2 low-fat protein portions
135 calories/ 38 mg. cholesterol/ 181 mg. sodium

TOSTADA

4 tortillas, toasted (whole or tortilla chips)
1 head lettuce, finely chopped
2 medium tomatoes, diced
1/2 cup Jones Cumin Dressing, page 128–129
1-1/2 cups cooked and diced chicken or turkey
1/2 cup (2 ounces) grated cheddar or Monterey Jack cheese
1/4 cup Mock Sour Cream, page 133
Chopped tomatoes for garnish

Toast the tortillas (or chips) and set aside. Combine the lettuce, 2 tomatoes and dressing and toss thoroughly. If using whole tortillas, place each one on a chilled dinner-size plate first and spoon the salad over the tortillas. If using tortilla chips, put the salad directly on the plates, garnishing later with the chips. Divide the chicken and cheese evenly over the salads. Top each with 1 tablespoon of Mock Sour Cream. Garnish with chopped tomatoes.

MAKES 4 servings. Each serving contains approximately:
1 starch portion/ 1/2 vegetable portion
1-3/4 low-fat protein portions/ 1/2 high-fat protein portion
227 calories/ 54 mg. cholesterol/ 286 mg. sodium

VARIATION: Serve bowls of chunky textured Gazpacho with the Tostadas to spoon over them as a salsa topping.

LAMB CHOPS DIJON

4 small thick lamb chops, all visible fat removed
1 lemon
Garlic salt
Freshly ground black pepper
1/3 cup Dijon-style mustard
4 teaspoons unprocessesd wheat bran
1 cup finely chopped fresh parsley

Preheat the oven to 500°. Place the lamb chops in a shallow baking dish and rub both sides of each chop with lemon. Then sprinkle both sides of each with garlic salt and black pepper.

Combine the mustard, bran and parsley and mix well. Cover each lamb chop with an equal amount of the parsley mixture, pressing it down firmly with your hands.

Put the lamb chops in the preheated oven for *4 minutes*. Then turn the oven *off* and *do not open* the door for 30 minutes.

NOTE: This is an ideal dinner entrée for busy people who give dinner parties. You can prepare the lamb chops many hours in advance or even a day ahead of time. Cover them tightly and refrigerate until 34 minutes before serving. (Even if you leave them in a little longer than 30 minutes after the oven is turned off the chops will not be over-cooked.) If you prefer lamb chops well-done, bake them for 5 minutes instead of 4 before turning off the oven. I prefer this recipe to lamb with mint jelly—and it doesn't contain any refined carbohydrates!

MAKES 4 servings. Each serving contains approximately:
2 low-fat protein portions/ 110 calories
56 mg. cholesterol/ 419 mg. sodium

TERIYAKI STEAK

1-3/4 cups salt-reduced soy sauce
3 tablespoons pure crystalline fructose
2 cloves garlic, crushed
1 tablespoon peeled and grated fresh ginger root
2 pounds flank steak, all visible fat removed

Combine all ingredients, except the flank steak, and store in the refrigerator for 1 day before using. Marinate the flank steak for 1–2 hours in the marinade before cooking, depending upon how strong you want the teriyaki flavor. Broil 3–5 minutes per side, depending on the thickness of the flank steak, for a rare teriyaki steak.

MAKES 8 servings. Each serving contains approximately:
2 low-fat protein portions/ 110 calories
85 mg. cholesterol/ 600 mg. sodium

BREADS AND OTHER STARCHES

CANYON RANCH BREAD

1-1/4 cups non-fat milk
1 tablespoon fresh lemon juice
1/4 cup finely chopped raisins
1 cup unprocessed wheat bran
1/4 cup pure crystalline fructose
1 tablespoon vanilla extract
1 egg, lightly beaten, or 1/4 cup liquid egg substitute
1-1/2 cups whole-wheat flour
2 teaspoons baking powder

Combine the milk and lemon juice in a large mixing bowl and mix well. Let stand for 5 minutes. Add the raisins, wheat bran, fructose and vanilla extract to the bowl and mix well. Cover and let stand for 30 minutes. Preheat the oven to 350°. Mix the egg or egg substitute into the bran mixture. Combine the whole-wheat flour and baking powder in a large bowl and mix well. Add the liquid ingredients to the dry ingredients and blend thoroughly.

Spray a standard-sized metal loaf pan with a non-stick spray. Transfer the batter to the pan and bake in the preheated oven for 1 hour, or until a wooden pick inserted in the center comes out clean. Remove the bread from the oven and place it on its side on a rack to cool.

When the bread is cool enough to handle, remove it from the pan and cool on a rack to room temperature. Wrap the cooled bread tightly in aluminum foil and refrigerate until cold before slicing.

To serve, slice the loaf in half lengthwise, then cut each half into 12 slices. Lightly spread each slice with corn oil margarine, if desired. Rewrap the bread in foil and reheat in a preheated 325° oven for 30 minutes.

MAKES 1 loaf (24 slices). Each slice contains approximately:
1/4 fruit portion/ 1/2 starch portion/ 45 calories
13 mg. cholesterol/ 10 mg. sodium

DILL BREAD

1 yeast cake or 1 package dry yeast (check date on package)
1/4 cup warm water
1 cup low-fat cottage cheese
4 teaspoons pure crystalline fructose
1/4 cup minced onion
1/4 teaspoon baking soda
1 egg, lightly beaten
2 tablespoons dried dill seed
1 teaspoon salt
2 cups whole-wheat flour

Soften the yeast in 1/4 cup warm water. Warm the cottage cheese in a saucepan. Add the yeast in the water to the warm cottage cheese. Add the fructose, minced onion, baking soda, beaten egg, dill seed and salt. Mix well. Add the sifted flour, a little at a time, mixing well. Cover and allow to stand at room temperature for several hours, or until doubled in bulk. Stir the dough until reduced to original size, and put it in a well-oiled, standard-sized metal loaf pan. Cover the loaf pan and again allow the dough to double in bulk. Bake in a 350° oven for 40 minutes.

This bread is delicious right from the oven. However, it's much easier to slice when cool. Wrap sliced bread in foil and store in the refrigerator until ready to use. Then warm in the oven before serving.

MAKES 1 loaf (18 slices). Each slice contains approximately:
1 starch portion/ 70 calories
15 mg. cholesterol/ 196 mg. sodium

SPROUTED WHEAT BERRY BREAD

1-1/2 cups wheat berries
2 cups water
Unprocessed wheat bran

Soak the wheat berries overnight in the water. Drain, rinse and drain again. Line the bottoms of 2 large glass baking dishes with damp cheesecloth (white paper towels may also be used). Spread the wheat berries evenly over the damp cheesecloth and cover with another layer of wet cheesecloth. Sprinkle at least twice a day for 3 days, keeping the berries damp but not wet.

On the third morning, remove the sprouts from the cheesecloth (or towels) and place in a food processor, a few at a time, grinding them into a doughlike consistency. Form the dough into a ball and roll in unprocessed wheat bran, lightly covering the entire outer surface of the ball. Flatten into a 5-inch round loaf and place on a non-stick baking pan or cookie sheet and bake in a preheated 250° oven 2 hours.

MAKES 1 round loaf 5 inches in diameter.
1/8 loaf contains approximately:
1-1/4 starch portions/ 88 calories/ 0 cholesterol/ 50 mg. sodium

VARIATION: Add grated orange rind or raisins to the dough ball.

WHOLE-WHEAT BREAD

1 cup non-fat milk, heated to luke warm (110° to 115°)
1 tablespoon freshly squeezed lemon juice
2 packages (2 tablespoons) active dry yeast (check date on package)
2 tablespoons pure crystalline fructose
1 egg, lightly beaten, or 1/2 cup liquid egg substitute
1/4 cup corn oil
1 teaspoon salt
3-1/4 cups whole-wheat flour
Unsalted butter or corn oil margarine, softened, for glazing (optional)

Combine the milk and lemon juice and mix well. Add the yeast and fructose and again mix well. Set aside out of a draft and allow to double in bulk. (This takes only a few minutes.) Combine the egg or egg substitute and corn oil and mix well. Add the yeast mixture to the egg-oil mixture, again mixing well. Combine the salt and flour. Add the flour, a little at a time, until thoroughly mixed. (You will have to knead the last 1/2 cup of flour in with your hands.)

Cover with a tea towel and allow to rise in a warm place until doubled in bulk, about 1-1/2 hours. Then punch down and knead on a floured board for 10 minutes, or until the dough is smooth and elastic.

Lightly rub the dough ball with butter or margarine, cover with a tea towel and allow to rise again until double in bulk, about 30 minutes. Knead the dough again briefly and form it into a loaf shape. Place the dough in a greased $9 \times 5 \times 3$-inch loaf pan, cover with a tea towel and allow to rise until nearly double in bulk, about 30 minutes.

While the bread is rising the third time, preheat the oven to 375°. Bake for 40 minutes or until it is a golden brown and sounds hollow when tapped. If you want to glaze the bread, rub the top of the loaf with a little butter or margarine 3 or 4 minutes before baking time is completed. Remove the bread from the oven, place it on its side for 5 minutes, then turn out on a rack and cool to room temperature. (The loaf is much easier to slice when it is cool. If you wish to serve the bread hot, slice it when cool, butter it if desired, wrap it in foil and reheat in the oven.)

MAKES 1 loaf (24 slices). 1 slice contains approximately:
1-1/2 starch portions/ 105 calories
13 mg. cholesterol/ 107 mg. sodium

LEMON ONION BULGUR

1-1/2 cups chicken stock
1/4 teaspoon salt
3/4 cup bulgur (cracked wheat)
1/2 medium onion, finely chopped
1-1/2 teaspoons freshly grated lemon rind

Bring the chicken stock and salt to a boil in a saucepan. Add the bulgur and chopped onion and bring back to a boil. Cover, reduce the heat to low and cook for 25 minutes. Remove the lid, add the grated lemon rind and mix thoroughly.

MAKES 4 (1/2-cup) servings. Each serving contains approximately:
1 starch portion/ 70 calories/ 0 cholesterol/ 200 mg. sodium

PASTA PRIMAVERA

1/2 cup peas
1/2 cup diced carrots
1 cup diced zucchini
1 cup diced yellow squash
1 large onion, peeled and diced
1 cup broccoli flowerets (small pieces)
8–10 cups water
1/2 pound whole-wheat spaghetti noodles (4 cups cooked)
2 teaspoons cornstarch
1 cup chicken stock
1/4 cup Parmesan cheese
1 small tomato, peeled and diced

Steam the vegetables until crisp-tender and set aside. Bring the water to a boil and add the spaghetti. Bring back to a boil and cook for 8–10 minutes or until it has a slight resilience (al dente). While the spaghetti is cooking, combine the cornstarch and a little of the chicken stock and mix until the cornstarch is completely dissolved. Combine the remaining chicken stock and bring to a boil. Reduce the heat and stir constantly until thickened. Drain the spaghetti thoroughly and put in a large bowl. Add the Parmesan cheese to the thickened chicken stock and mix thoroughly. Pour over the drained spaghetti, tossing thoroughly.

Add the steamed vegetables and again toss thoroughly. Divide the vegetable-pasta mixture in 4 servings. Garnish each serving with diced tomatoes.

MAKES 4 (2-cup) servings. Each serving contains approximately:
2 vegetable portions/ 1 starch portion
1/4 medium-fat protein portion/ 139 calories
8 mg. cholesterol/ 114 mg. sodium

VEGETARIAN VARIATION: Substitute non-fat milk for chicken stock.
LOW-FAT COTTAGE CHEESE VARIATION: Add 1-1/2 cups low-fat cottage cheese or partially skimmed ricotta cheese with the Parmesan.
NOTE: This is a good recipe for using lots of leftover steamed vegetables—a colorful combination makes a more attractive presentation.

TOASTED CHOW MEIN NOODLES

4 ounces whole-wheat spaghetti
Water to cover

Break the spaghetti into 3-inch pieces for easier handling. Cover with water and boil for 15 minutes. Drain thoroughly, using a colander. Place on a large cookie sheet in the oven and bake at 375° for an hour, turning frequently to toast evenly.

MAKES 4 servings (approximately 1 cup each).
Each serving contains approximately:
1 starch portion/ 70 calories/ 0 cholesterol/ 3 mg. sodium

OVERBAKED POTATOES

2 large baking potatoes

Preheat the oven to 450°. Wash the potatoes well. Dry thoroughly and pierce them several times with a fork. Place them in the center of the preheated 450° oven and bake for 2 hours. Remove from the oven and cut lengthwise and then across the middle, almost through the potatoes. The shells will be very crisp and thick and will not squeeze easily. Open the potatoes and mash the inside pulp as best you can with a fork.

MAKES 2 servings. Each serving contains approximately:
2 starch portions/ 140 calories/ 0 cholesterol/ 4 mg. sodium

NOTE: Recently, when I was discussing baked potatoes with James Beard, he asked me if I had ever eaten a potato baked for 2 hours at 450°. I thought I had misunderstood him and asked again how long and at what temperature. He assured me that the result was both unusual and delicious. The potato itself has a very thick, crunchy outer shell, almost like a pastry shell. The inside has a rich, creamy texture. He likes it best served only with freshly ground black pepper. I do too, but I also like it served with Mustard Dip, page 131.

STUFFED BAKED POTATO

2 small baking potatoes
1 medium onion, finely chopped
1/4 cup chicken stock
1/2 cup low-fat cottage cheese
2 tablespoons chopped chives or green onion tops

Wash the potatoes well. Pierce with a fork and bake at 400° for 1 hour. Cut a very thin slice from the top of each potato. Remove the pulp from the potato, being careful not to tear the shell. Mash the potato pulp and set aside in a covered bowl. Keep the shells warm.

Sauté the onion in the chicken stock until clear and tender. Add the mashed potato and cottage cheese and mix well and heat thoroughly. Stuff the potato mixture back into the warm shells. They will be heaping way over the top. To serve, sprinkle each potato with 1 tablespoon of chopped chives or green onion tops. If you have prepared them in advance, heat in a 350° oven for 10 to 15 minutes, or until hot, before adding the chopped chives.

MAKES 2 servings. Each serving contains approximately:
1 starch portion/ 1/2 vegetable portion
1 low-fat protein protion/ 138 calories
3 mg. cholesterol/ 266 mg. sodium

CANYON RANCH STUFT SPUD: Add 2 tablespoons grated Parmesan with the cottage cheese. I developed this recipe for the Canyon Ranch Vacation/Fitness Resort in Tucson, Arizona, where it has become one of the more popular luncheon entrées. It is served with a green salad, and fresh fruit for dessert. This adds 1/4 medium-fat protein portion/ 19 calories/ 4 mg. cholesterol/ 41 mg. sodium.

POWERFUL PORRIDGE
(LIFETIME)

1 cup unprocessed wheat bran
2 cups rolled oats
1/2 cup chopped almonds
1 cup chopped dried prunes
1/2 cup raisins
1 teaspoon ground cinnamon
4 cups water

Combine all dry ingredients in a mixing bowl and mix well. Add the water, mix well, cover and refrigerate overnight before serving. It is even better to wait 2 or 3 days before serving.

    Serve Powerful Porridge cold. I like it best plain or with a few slices of banana on top. My family likes it better with milk or yogurt on it. It is also good with ricotta or cottage cheese. For Basic Weight-Loss Diet, omit the almonds.

MAKES 6 cups. 1/2 cup contains approximately:
1-1/2 fruit portions/ 1 starch portion/ 1/2 fat portion
153 calories/ 0 cholesterol/ Tr. sodium

TABBOULI
(LEBANESE SALAD)

1 cup uncooked bulgur (cracked wheat)
Hot water to cover bulgur
1/4 cup fresh lemon juice
1/2 teaspoon salt
1/4 teaspoon freshly ground black pepper
1 clove garlic, minced
1 tablespoon water
2 tomatoes, diced
1 cup chopped green onions
1 cup minced fresh parsley
1/2 cup minced fresh mint leaves
24 small Romaine lettuce leaves

Soak the bulgur in hot water for 30 minutes.

While the bulgur is soaking, make the dressing. Combine the lemon juice and salt and stir until the salt has dissolved. Add the pepper, garlic and water and mix well. Put the dressing in a jar with a tightly fitted lid and shake vigorously for 30 seconds. Set aside.

Drain the bulgur thoroughly. Add the tomato, parsley, green onions and mint leaves to the bulgur. Add the dressing and toss thoroughly. Chill well.

Serve on chilled salad plates with each serving surrounded by 3 Romaine leaves. Traditionally this salad is eaten by scooping it onto the lettuce leaves.

MAKES 8 servings. Each serving contains approximately:
3/4 starch portion/ 1/2 vegetable portion
66 calories/ 0 cholesterol/ 138 mg. sodium

WILD RICE PILAF

3/4 cup wild rice (4 ounces)
1-1/2 cups chicken stock
1-1/2 teaspoons soy sauce
1 teaspoon dried thyme, crushed, using a mortar and pestle
1/4 cup chicken stock
1 medium onion, chopped
1 celery stalk without leaves, chopped

Combine the wild rice, chicken stock, soy sauce and thyme in a saucepan. Bring to a boil, reduce the heat, cover and simmer for 30 to 35 minutes or until all the liquid is absorbed and the rice is fluffy. Remove from the heat and set aside.

Heat the 1/4 cup chicken stock in a skillet and add the chopped onion and celery. Sauté over medium heat until the onion is clear and tender. Combine cooked rice, cooked onion and celery and mix well.

MAKES 6 (1/2-cup) servings (3 cups). 1/2 cup contains approximately:
1 starch portion/ 70 calories/ 0 cholesterol/ 158 mg. sodium

VARIATION: Substitute brown rice for wild rice.
NOTE: If using salted chicken stock (or commercial chicken broth), only use 1 teaspoon of soy sauce.

DESSERTS AND FRUITS

BAKED APPLES

6 small green cooking apples
2 cups water
2 teaspoons vanilla extract
1/2 teaspoon ground cinnamon
1/2 cup pure crystalline fructose

Preheat the oven to 350°. Wash and core the apples. Remove the peel from the top third of each apple. Arrange the apples in a baking dish just large enough to hold them snugly.

In a saucepan, bring the water, vanilla extract, cinnamon and fructose to a boil and pour over the apples. Bake for 1 hour or until the apples can be easily pierced with a fork, basting frequently as they cook. When the apples are done, remove them from the oven and let cool in the sauce. They are good served hot or cold.

MAKES 6 servings. Each serving contains approximately:
2 fruit portions/ 80 calories/ 0 cholesterol/ 1 mg. sodium

BANANA SORBET

2 ripe bananas, thinly sliced
1 teaspoon freshly grated orange peel for garnish
Fresh mint sprigs for garnish (optional)

Put the sliced bananas in a plastic bag in the freezer. When the bananas are completely frozen and hard, put them in a blender container or food processor with a metal blade, a few at a time, and blend until smooth. Spoon the frozen puréed bananasinto 4 sherbet glasses and garnish with freshly grated orange peel and fresh mint.

MAKES 4 servings. Each serving contains approximately:
1 fruit portion/ 40 calories/ 0 cholesterol/ 1 mg. sodium

FRESH FRUIT COMPOTE

3/4 cup plain non-fat yogurt
1 small banana, sliced
1 small orange, diced
1 cup diced fresh pineapple or pineapple chunks
packed in natural juice, drained

Put the yogurt and banana in a blender and blend until smooth. Set aside. Combine the diced oranges and pineapple and serve 1/3 cup in each consommé cup with 1/4 cup of the sauce over the top of each serving. Any other fresh fruit may be substituted for the orange and pineapple.

MAKES 4 servings. Each serving contains approximately:
1-1/4 fruit portions/ 1/4 non-fat milk portion
70 calories/ 3 mg. cholesterol/ 23 mg. sodium

FROZEN GRAPES

Ripe grapes

Divide the grapes into small bunches and place in the freezer for several hours or until very hard. To serve, place the frozen grape bunches in sherbet dishes, small bowls or plates. Frozen grapes are a wonderful low-calorie dessert, which must be eaten slowly out of necessity!

12 large grapes or 20 Thompson seedless grapes
contain approximately:
1 fruit portion/ 40 calories/ 0 cholesterol/ 2 mg. sodium

JONES APPLE BUTTER

6 medium apples (2 pounds), peeled, cored and thinly sliced (6 cups)
1 cup unsweetened apple juice
1 teaspoon ground cinnamon
1/2 teaspoon ground allspice
1/4 teaspoon ground cloves

Combine all of the ingredients in a large saucepan and bring to a boil. Reduce the heat and simmer, uncovered, for 12 minutes, stirring occasionally. Remove from the heat and cool slightly.

Place the mixture in a blender container and blend until smooth. Store, covered, in the refrigerator.

MAKES 3 cups. 1/4 cup contains approximately:
1 fruit portion/ 40 calories/ 0 cholesterol/ 1 mg. sodium

NOTE: 1 teaspoon contains less than 4 calories and may be used sparingly on the Food Lover's Basic Diet.

MEDITERRANEAN MELON BALLS

1/3 cup unsweetened apple juice
1 teaspoon arrowroot
1/4 teaspoon ground aniseed
2 cups melon balls (1 medium cantaloupe)

Combine the apple juice and arrowroot in a saucepan and stir until the arrowroot is completely dissolved. Add the aniseed and mix thoroughly. Slowly bring the mixture to a boil and simmer until slightly thickened. Remove the pan from the heat and cool to room temperature. Combine the sauce with the melon balls and refrigerate until chilled before serving.

MAKES 2 cups melon balls. 1/2 cup contains approximately:
1-1/4 fruit portions/ 50 calories/ 0 cholesterol/ 11 mg. sodium

MINTED PINEAPPLE

1 20-ounce can crushed pineapple in natural juice, undrained
1/4 teaspoon mint extract

Combine the crushed pineapple and mint extract and refrigerate, covered, for 1 hour before serving.

MAKES 8 servings (scant 1/3 cup each).
Each serving contains approximately:
1 fruit portion/ 40 calories/ 0 cholesterol/ 1 mg. sodium

PEACHES "AMARETTO"

1/2 cup non-fat milk
1-1/2 teaspoons cornstarch
1-1/2 teaspoons pure crystalline fructose
3/4 teaspoon vanilla extract
1/4 teaspoon almond extract
1 egg white at room temperature
4 medium peaches, peeled, pitted and sliced (when fresh peaches are
not available, peaches canned in water or natural juice may be used)

Put the milk in a saucepan. Add the cornstarch and fructose and stir until the cornstarch is thoroughly dissolved. Place the pan on low heat and slowly bring to a boil. Simmer, stirring constantly with a wire whisk, until slightly thickened. Remove the pan from the heat and allow to cool to room temperature. Add the vanilla extract and the almond extract and mix thoroughly. Beat the egg white until stiff but not dry and fold into the sauce. Divide the sliced peaches into 4 sherbet glasses or serving dishes and spoon an equal amount of the sauce over each serving.

MAKES 4 servings. Each serving contains approximately:
1 fruit portion/ 1/8 non-fat milk portion
50 calories/ Tr. cholesterol/ 26 mg. sodium

PINEAPPLE BOATS WITH COCONUT SAUCE

2 fresh pineapples
2 cups Coconut Sauce, page 125
Ground cinnamon

Cut the pineapples lengthwise into quarters, carefully cutting through the green leaves at the top to leave a section of leaves on each quarter. Using a very small, sharp paring knife, carefully cut the fruit from its shell. It is necessary to cut down both sides of the pineapple sections, beginning at the corners, to do this. Cut off the hard core section at the top of each pineapple quarter and discard it. Cut each pineapple quarter as it rests on its shell in half lengthwise, then cut it horizontally into bite-sized pieces. To serve, top each pineapple boat with 1/4 cup of Coconut Sauce and sprinkle lightly with cinnamon.

MAKES 8 servings. Each serving contains approximately:
1 fruit portion/ 1/4 non-fat milk portion
60 calories/ 2 mg. cholesterol/ 32 mg. sodium

VARIATION: Use 1/2 cup drained pineapple chunks packed in natural juice instead of fresh pineapple for each serving. Serve in sherbet glasses and pour the sauce over the top of each serving.

POACHED PEARS IN SAUTERNE SAUCE

4 ripe, firm pears (Bartletts are best)
4 cups water
1 tablespoon vanilla extract
1 teaspoon rum extract
1/3 cup pure crystalline fructose
1 teaspoon ground cinnamon
1 cup Sauterne Sauce, page 126
Ground nutmeg for garnish

Peel the pears carefully, leaving the stems on them. With an apple corer, remove the core from the end opposite the stem. Put the water, vanilla, rum extract, fructose and cinnamon in a saucepan and bring to a boil.

Reduce the heat and simmer for 10 minutes. Place the pears in the simmering water and cook, turning frequently, about 10 minutes or until easily pierced with a fork, but not soft. Remove the pears from the heat and let cool to room temperature. Cover and refrigerate all day or overnight in the poaching liquid. Place each pear on a plate or in a shallow bowl and spoon 2 tablespoons of Sauterne Sauce over the top. Then sprinkle each serving with a touch of nutmeg. This is a delicious dessert. The sweet pear coupled with the tangy sauce makes an unusual combination. It is also good served as a side dish with poultry in the place of a fruit salad.

MAKES 4 servings. Each serving contains approximately:
2-1/2 fruit portions/ 1/4 non-fat milk portion
120 calories/ 3 mg. cholesterol/ 139 mg. sodium

STRAWBERRIES ROMANOFF

1/2 cup non-fat milk
1-1/2 teaspoons cornstarch
1 tablespoon pure crystalline fructose
3/4 teaspoon vanilla extract
1 tablespoon Grand Marnier
1 egg white, at room temperature
1/8 teaspoon cream of tartar
2 cups sliced fresh strawberries
4 whole strawberries

Put the milk in a saucepan. Add the cornstarch and fructose and stir until the cornstarch is thoroughly dissolved. Place the pan on low heat and bring to a boil. Simmer, stirring constantly with a wire whisk, until slightly thickened. Remove from heat and cool to room temperature.

Add the vanilla extract and Grand Marnier to the cooled sauce and mix well. Combine the egg white and cream of tartar and beat until stiff but not dry. Fold the beaten egg white into the sauce, then combine the sauce and the sliced strawberries and mix well. Divide evenly into 4 sherbet glasses. Place a whole strawberry on top of each serving for garnish.

MAKES 4 servings. Each serving contains approximately:
1 fruit portion/ 1/4 low-fat protein portion
1/8 non-fat milk portion/ 64 calories
Tr. cholesterol/ 29 mg. sodium

SHERRIED GRAPES

1 pound large purple grapes
1 cup sherry

Wash the grapes thoroughly and pat dry. Divide the grapes into 8 small bunches. Cut a criss-cross at the bottom of each grape and carefully remove the seeds, keeping the bunches intact. Put the 8 bunches of seeded grapes in a large bowl and pour the sherry over them. Cover and refrigerate for several hours before serving, turning the grapes from time to time so that they marinate evenly.

MAKES 8 servings. Each serving contains approximately:
1 fruit portion/ 40 calories/ 0 cholesterol/ 2 mg. sodium

CHEESECAKE (LIFETIME)

2 teaspoons corn oil margarine
4 graham cracker squares
2 cups low-fat cottage cheese
1/4 cup pure crystalline fructose
2 teaspoons vanilla extract
1 teaspoon freshly grated lemon rind
1 teaspoon fresh lemon juice

TOPPING:
3/4 cup sour cream
2 tablespoons pure crystalline fructose
1-1/2 teaspoons vanilla extract

Preheat oven to 375°. Rub 2 teaspoons margarine evenly over entire surface of a 9-inch pie plate. Put the 4 graham cracker squares in a plastic bag and roll them with a rolling pin until they are fine crumbs. Sprinkle the crumbs evenly over the greased pie plate, pressing them down with your fingertips to make certain they stick to the surface.

Put the cottage cheese, fructose, vanilla extract, lemon rind and lemon juice in a blender container and blend until smooth. Pour the cottage cheese mixture into the graham cracker shell, spreading it evenly. Place in the center of the preheated oven and cook for 15 minutes.

While the cake is baking, combine all of the topping ingredients in a mixing bowl and mix thoroughly. Remove the cheesecake from the oven and spread the topping evenly over the top. Place the cake back in the oven and continue baking for 10 minutes. Cool to room temperature on a wire rack and refrigerate until chilled before serving.

MAKES 16 servings. Each serving contains approximately:
1/2 low-fat protein portion/ 1/2 fruit portion/ 1/2 fat portion
71 calories/ 9 mg. cholesterol/ 138 mg. sodium

BLUEBERRY CHEESECAKE: Add 1 cup frozen unsweetened blueberries, unthawed, to the topping ingredients and mix thoroughly. This will not increase the fruit portion or calories appreciably when you cut the cheesecake into 16 servings.

HOLIDAY PUMPKIN CREAM

1 cup canned pumpkin
1 cup partially skimmed ricotta cheese
2 tablespoons pure crystalline fructose
1 teaspoon ground cinnamon
1/2 teaspoon ground allspice
1/4 teaspoon ground ginger
2 teaspoons vanilla extract

Combine all ingredients in a blender container and blend until completely smooth. Spoon into a bowl. Cover and refrigerate for several hours before serving. To serve, use a 4-ounce (1/2-cup) ice cream scoop and place 1 pumpkin cream ball in each of 4 sherbet glasses.

MAKES 4 servings (2 cups). Each serving contains approximately:
1/4 starch portion/ 1/2 low-fat protein portion/ 66 calories
5 mg. cholesterol/ 13 mg. sodium

JELLED FRUIT CAKE

1 envelope (1 tablespoon) unflavored gelatin
2 tablespoons cold water
1/4 cup boiling water
1/2 cup non-fat milk
1/2 cup unsweetened applesauce
1/2 cup raisins
1 tablespoon pure crystalline fructose
1/2 teaspoon ground cinnamon
1/4 teaspoon ground allspice
1/8 teaspoon carob powder or unsweetened cocoa
1 teaspoon vanilla extract
1 8-ounce can crushed pineapple packed in natural juice, well drained
1/2 cup chopped walnuts

Soften the gelatin in the cold water for 5 minutes. Add the boiling water and stir until the gelatin is completely dissolved. Pour the gelatin mixture and all of the ingredients, except the crushed pineapple and walnuts, into a blender container. Blend until mixed thoroughly and raisins are coarsely chopped. Pour the blended mixture into a bowl and add the crushed pineapple. Mix thoroughly. Pour the mixture into an oiled 8-inch cake pan. Refrigerate until firm, several hours or overnight.

Before serving, preheat the oven to 350°. Place the walnuts on a baking sheet in the center of the preheated oven for 8 to 10 minutes, or until golden brown. Watch them carefully, as they burn easily. Remove the jelled fruit cake from the refrigerator and invert on a cake plate. Turn right side up and sprinkle the toasted walnuts evenly over the top of the cake.

MAKES 8 servings. Each serving contains approximately:
1 fruit portion/ 1/4 fat portion/ 52 calories
Tr. cholesterol/ 12 mg. sodium

BEVERAGES

BLOODY SHAME
(BLOODY MARY WITHOUT VODKA)

1 teaspoon fresh lime juice
1/2 teaspoon Worcestershire sauce
1/4 teaspoon seasoned salt
Dash freshly ground pepper
1 cup V-8 juice or tomato juice
Dash Tabasco (optional)

Mix the lime juice, Worcestershire sauce, seasoned salt and pepper together until the salt is dissolved. Add V-8 or tomato juice and mix. Add Tabasco if desired. Pour over ice and garnish with a celery stick for a stirrer.

MAKES 2 servings. Each serving contains approximately:
1 vegetable portion/ 25 calories/ 0 cholesterol
661 mg. sodium (V-8 juice)/ 492 mg. sodium (regular tomato juice)
285 mg. sodium (unsalted V-8 juice)
274 mg. sodium (unsalted tomato juice)

COUNTERFEIT COCKTAIL

Perrier water or soda water (enough to fill a tall glass)
Ice cubes
1/2 fresh lime
Dash of Angostura bitters

Pour the soda water over ice in a tall glass. Add the juice of the lime and a dash of bitters. Stir and serve.
MAKES 1 serving.
0 cholesterol/ Tr. sodium/ Calories negligible

FAKE MARGARITA

1-1/2 cups soda water or Perrier water
2 tablespoons fresh lime juice
1 tablespoon pure crystalline fructose
1 egg white (dip the egg in boiling water
for 30 seconds before breaking)
1/2 cup crushed ice
Coarse salt (optional)
Ice cubes
Lime slices for garnish

Pour the soda water into a blender container. Add the lime juice, fructose, egg white and crushed ice and blend until frothy. Rub lime around the rims of 4 chilled glasses. Dip the rim of each glass into the salt (optional). Fill each glass with ice cubes and then fill with the frothy margarita mixture and garnish each with a slice of lime.

MAKES 4 servings. Each serving contains approximately:
1/4 fruit portion/ 10 calories
0 cholesterol/ 42 mg. sodium (without the coarse salt!)

PINA COLADA PUNCH

2 cups non-fat milk
2 cups unsweetened pineapple juice
1 tablespoon vanilla extract
2 tablespoons pure crystalline fructose

Place all of the ingredients in a blender container and blend until frothy.

MAKES 4 (1-cup) servings. Each serving contains approximately:
2 fruit portions/ 1/2 non-fat milk portion/ 120 calories
2 mg. cholesterol/ 65 mg. sodium

SOY MILK

3/4 cup soy powder
4 cups water

Combine the soy powder and 1 cup of the water in a saucepan and stir into a paste. Add the remaining water and bring to a boil. Reduce the heat and simmer for 3–5 minutes. Refrigerate (may be served hot or cold).

MAKES 4 cups. 1 cup contains approximately:
1 non-fat milk portion/ 80 calories/ 0 cholesterol/ 2 mg. sodium

USING HERBS AND SPICES   ·

We have only four basic tastes. They are, in order, from the tip of the tongue back: sweet, salt, sour and bitter. All other "tastes" are actually smells. If you don't believe me, hold your nose the next time you eat and you will find that you don't "taste" anything!

Because our sense of smell is so important to the flavor of our food, herbs and spices can play a very important role in making foods taste better. Also by using herbs and spices imaginatively, you can create a new and exciting flavor range in your cooking and baking.

Fresh herbs and spices are wonderful; they always add a glamorous touch as well as a delightful flavor. Try growing at least some of your own herbs if you possibly can. Having your own herb garden is lots of fun, especially when you can go right outside your back door or to your window sill and pick the herbs. Always use fresh parsley. Dried parsley, in my opinion, tastes exactly like hay, smells badly and tends to ruin rather than enhance flavor.

When using dry herbs and spices, always grind them well, using a mortar and pestle, before adding them to your recipe. This is very important because it releases their aromatic qualities and thus increases the strength of flavor. You can tell when you have ground them enough because the odor of the herb or spice will be at least three times as strong.

It is not necessary to grind already-ground spices, such as curry powder, ground ginger, nutmeg and cinnamon.

It is fun to be adventuresome when seasoning the foods you prepare. The following list of herbs and spices gives suggestions for all of their usual uses, as well as some rather unusual ones. Not only will learning to use more herbs and spices in your cooking add a whole new flavor dimension to your menus, it will also help you get started on the road to much healthier cooking in general. As you learned in the section on sodium, the best way to reduce the amount of salt in a recipe without noticing it is to add more (up to three times as much) of an herb or spice as you normally would. This is because salt, a basic taste, sharpens flavors. It cannot create a flavor since flavors (other than the four basic tastes) rely strictly on a sense of smell. Obviously the more flavor or taste a food has, the less it needs sharpening.

USES FOR HERBS & SPICES

ALLSPICE Fruit, sweet potatoes, squash, eggs, fish, pot roast

ANISE Cheese, beverages, cookies, cakes, breads, fish, stew, fruit dishes

BASIL All vegetables, fish, meat and poultry, egg dishes, sauces and salad dressings, all Italian dishes in combination with oregano

BAY LEAF Roasts, stews, soups, marinades, poultry dressings, chowders

CARDAMOM Fruit soups, squash, baked goods, sweet potatoes

CAYENNE PEPPER Sauces, vegetables, cheese, eggs, fish, chicken, pizza, spaghetti, meat dishes

CELERY SEED Soups, stews, meat loaf, egg dishes, breads, rolls, stuffings, potato salad, tomatoes, many other vegetables

CHILI POWDER Corn, bean casseroles, cheese, marinades, chicken, meat loaf, stews, egg dishes, tomato or barbecue sauces, dips

CINNAMON Lamb or beef stews, roast lamb, chicken, pork, ham, beverages, bakery products, fruits

CLOVES Glazed pork or beef, tomatoes, sweet potatoes, carrots, green beans, marinades for meats, pot roast, meat sauces, stuffings, fish, baked goods, fruits and for studding ham

CORIANDER Meat and poultry, stuffing, curry sauces, fruit, barbecue sauce, fruit salads, custards, marinated bean salads

CUMIN Chili, omelets, salad dressings

CURRY POWDER Curried beef, poultry and fish dishes, eggs, dried beans, fruit, dips, breads, salad dressings and marinades

DILL SEED AND DILL WEED Sauces, green beans, egg dishes, fish, chicken, breads

FENNEL Sauerkraut, breads, cakes, cookies, egg dishes, fish, stews, marinades for meats, vegetables, cheese, baked or stewed apples

GARLIC Meat, poultry and fish, stews, marinades, tomato dishes, soups, dips, sauces, salads, salad dressings, etc.!

GINGER Baked or stewed fruits, vegetables, baked goods, poultry, fish and meat, beverages, soups, Oriental dishes of all types

JUNIPER BERRIES Venison, game or rabbit, stew, hot or cold drinks

MACE Fruits, meat loaf, fish, poultry, chowder, vegetables

MARJORAM Soups, breads, egg dishes, spaghetti, pizza, broccoli, mushrooms, squash, peas, cauliflower, carrots, tomato dishes, meat, poultry and fish

MINT Sauces for lamb and poultry, punches, tea, sauces for desserts, vegetables

DRY MUSTARD Vegetables, fish, meat and poultry, salad dressings, egg and cheese dishes

MUSTARD SEED Corned beef, cole slaw, potato salad, boiled cabbage, pickles, sauerkraut

NUTMEG Hot beverages, puddings, fish, meat and poultry, fruits, baked goods, eggs, vegetables, pickles

ONION POWDER Breads, egg dishes, rice dishes, cheese dishes, stuffing, vegetables, salads, fish, meat and poultry, stews, soups, dips

OREGANO Fish, meat and poultry, all vegetables, stuffings, cheese dishes, egg dishes, barbecue sauce, chili con carne, pizza, sauces for pasta, tomatoes

PAPRIKA Fish, meat and poultry, egg dishes, cheese dishes, to add color to colorless vegetables, sprinkled on casseroles for garnish

PARSLEY For garnish on many dishes, salads, broiled meat, fish and poultry, soups, cole slaw, breads, tomato and meat sauces

PEPPER (BLACK) Fish, meat, poultry, eggs, vegetables, pickles, etc.

PEPPER (RED) Barbecued beef or pork, tamale pie, dips, curried dishes, spaghetti sauce, vegetables, poultry, pickles, sauces, cheese dishes, soups, meat

PEPPER (WHITE) Vegetables, white or light meats, poultry and fish

POULTRY SEASONING Stuffings, poultry, veal, meat loaf, chicken soup

ROSEMARY Soups, stews, marinades, potatoes, cauliflower, spinach, mushrooms, turnips, fruits, breads, fish, meat and poultry

SAFFRON Chicken, seafood, rice

SAGE Stuffings for meat, fish and poultry, sauces, soups, chowders, marinades, onions, tomatoes, cheese and egg dishes

SAVORY Tomatoes and seafood

TARRAGON Casseroles, marinades, sauces and salad dressings, egg dishes, fish, meat and poultry

THYME Fish, meat and poultry, vegetables, rice

TURMERIC Chutney, pickles, rice dishes, egg dishes, curried meat, fish and poultry, breads, cakes

KITCHEN VOCABULARY

BAKE Cook in heated oven.

BARBECUE Cook over hot coals.

BASTE Spoon liquid over food while it is cooking as directed, or use a baster.

BEAT Using egg beater or electric mixer, beat to add air and increase volume.

BLANCH Dip quickly into boiling water. Usually refers to fruits and vegetables. When blanching nuts, cover shelled nuts with cold water and bring to a boil. Remove from heat and drain. Slip skins from nuts.

BLEND Combine two or more ingredients well; often used when referring to an electric blender.

BLEND UNTIL FROTHY Blend until foamy and the volume is almost doubled by the addition of air.

BOIL Cook food in liquid in which bubbles constantly rise to the surface and break. At sea level, water boils at 212°F.

BONE Remove all bones; usually refers to roasts and poultry.

BRAISE Brown meat well on all sides, then add a small amount of water or other liquid. Cover and simmer over low heat or place in a moderate oven

and cook until tender or as recipe directs.

BROIL Cook under broiler at designated distance from heat.

BROWN Brown in oven under a broiler or in a heavy iron skillet to desired color.

CHILL Place in refrigerator until cold.

CHOP Using a large chopping knife, hold point end down with one hand and use the other hand to chop. There are chopping devices available in most appliance and hardware stores.

COARSELY CHOP Chop in pieces approximately 1/2-inch square.

COAT Using a sifter, sprinkle ingredient with flour, cornmeal, etc., until coated. Or roll in flour or shake in a paper bag until coated.

CODDLE Usually refers to eggs. When a raw egg is called for in a recipe such as eggnog, Caesar salad, etc., put the egg in boiling water for 30 seconds before using it. The reason for coddling the egg is that avedin, a component of raw egg whites, is believed to block the absorption of biotin, one of the water-soluble vitamins. Avedin is extremely sensitive to heat and coddling the egg inactivates the avedin.

COOL Allow to stand at room temperature until no longer warm to the touch.

CORE Remove core from fruits such as pears and apples.

COVER TIGHTLY Seal so that steam cannot escape.

CREAM With a spoon, rub against sides of bowl until creamy. A pastry blender may also be used.

CRUMBLE Crush with your hands or a fork into crumblings.

CRUSH Crush dry herbs with a mortar and pestle before using.

CUBE Cut into cube-shaped pieces approximately 1 inch or specified size.

DEEP FRY Use a deep-fat fryer and add enough oil to cover food to be cooked. If temperature is given in the recipe, a deep-fat frying thermometer will be needed.

DICE Cut into 1/4-inch cubes or smaller.

DISSOLVE Mix dry ingredients with liquid until no longer visible in the solution.

DOT Scatter in small bits over surface of food, actually "sprinkling." Usually refers to butter or margarine.

DREDGE Sprinkle lightly with flour, or coat with flour.

FILLET Remove all bones; usually refers to fish.

FINELY CHOP Chop in pieces approximately 1/4-inch square.

FOLD IN Using a rubber spatula or spoon in a circular motion coming across the bottom, fold the bottom of a mixture over the top. Repeat slowly until mixture is folded in as indicated in the recipe.

FORK-TENDER When food can be easily pierced with a fork.

FRY Cook in a small amount of oil in a skillet.

GRATE Rub the surface to be grated on grater for desired-size particles. Finely grated and coarsely grated foods require two different size graters.

GREASE Rub lightly with margarine, corn oil, etc.

GRIND Use a food chopper or grinder.

JULIENNE CUT Cut in strips approximately 1/4 inch by 2 inches.

KNEAD Usually refers to bread dough. After mixing dough according to recipe, place on a floured surface, flatten ball of dough with floured hands and fold it toward you. With the heels of your hands, press down and flatten again. Continue doing this until dough is smooth and satiny, or as recipe directs.

MARINATE Allow mixture to stand in marinade for length of time indicated in recipe.

MASH Potatoes and many other cooked vegetables can be mashed using a potato masher, or brought to the same consistency in an electric blender or mixer.

MINCE Chop as fine as gravel.

PAN BROIL Cook in ungreased or cured hot skillet, pouring off fat as it accumulates.

PARBOIL Boil in water or other liquid until partially cooked. This usually precedes another method of cooking.

PARE Using a knife, remove the outer covering of foods such as apples and peaches.

PEEL Remove outer covering of foods such as oranges, lemons and bananas.

PIT Remove the pit or seed from fruits such as peaches and plums.

POACH Cook for a short time in simmering liquid.

PREHEAT Set oven to desired temperature. Wait until temperature is reached before baking.

PRESS Usually refers to garlic when using a garlic press.

ROAST To bake meat or poultry.

SAUTÉ Cook in small amount of hot oil in a skillet.

SCALD Heat to just under the boiling point when tiny bubbles begin to form on the sides of the pan. This is also often called "bring to a boiling point."

SCORE Using a knife, make shallow cuts or slits on surface of a food.

SCRAPE Scrape to remove outer skin on foods such as carrots and parsnips, or scrape to produce juice in foods such as onions.

SEAR Brown surface rapidly over high heat in a hot skillet.

SEED Completely remove small seeds from such foods as tomatoes, cucumbers and bell peppers.

SHRED Slice thinly in two directions, or use a shredder.

SIFT Put flour, sugar, etc., through a flour sifter or sieve.

SIMMER Cook just below boiling point (about 185°F at sea level).

SINGE Usually refers to poultry. Hold over flame to burn off all feathers or hairs.

SKEWER Hold together with metal or wooden skewers, or spear chunks of meat/vegetables on wooden skewers, as for shish kabob.

SKIN Remove skin of such foods as chicken; sometimes used when referring to onions.

SLICE Using a sharp knife, slice through evenly to specified thickness.

SNIP Cut into small pieces using scissors or kitchen shears.

SPRINKLE Just as the word implies, sprinkle, using your fingers.

STEAM Cook food over boiling water, using either a steamer or a large kettle with a rack placed in the bottom to hold the pan or dish of food above the boiling water.

STEEP Allow to stand in hot liquid.

STIFF BUT NOT DRY This term is often used for egg whites and means they should form soft, well-defined peaks but not be beaten to the point where the peaks look as though they will break.

STIFFLY BEATEN Beat until mixture stands in stiff peaks.

STIR Mix with a wooden spoon in a circular motion until all ingredients are well blended.

THICKEN Mix a thickening agent such as arrowroot, cornstarch, flour, etc., with a small amount of liquid to be thickened, then add slowly to the hot liquid, stirring constantly. Cook until slightly thickened or until mixture coats a metal spoon.

THINLY SLICE Using the slicing side of a four-sided grater, slice vegetables such as cucumbers and onions.

TOAST Brown in a toaster, oven or under a broiler. Nuts, seeds or coconut may be toasted in a 350° oven until desired color is attained. Or, place under a broiler and watch carefully, as they burn quickly.

TOSS Mix from both sides in an under-and-over motion toward the center, using two spoons or a fork and spoon; usually refers to salads.

WHIP Beat rapidly with fork, whisk, egg beater or electric mixer to add air and increase volume of mixture.

WHISK Stir, beat or fold using a wire whisk.

FOOD LISTS AND EQUIVALENTS

FOOD PORTION CATEGORIES

The following table summarizes the calorie and nutritional content of each food portion category, including the percentage of carbohydrate, protein and fat calories in each. Because the Exchange Diet of the American Diabetes Association, upon which this is based, rounds off numbers to the nearest whole digit ending in either "0" or "5" to make it easier for laypersons to compute their calorie intake, the percentages in a category will seldom total exactly 100 percent. The percentages are primarily to show you the importance of concentrating on fruits, vegetables, starches (complex carbohydrates), *low-fat* proteins and *non-fat* milk when trying to lose or maintain weight. Fat will make you *fat* faster!

Portion sizes are shown on the following Food Lists.

FOOD PORTION CATEGORY (For One Food Portion)	CALORIES	CARBOHYDRATE Grams x4 Calories		PROTEIN Grams x4 Calories		FAT Grams x9 Calories	
Fruit	40	10	40(100%)				
Vegetable	25	5	20 (80%)	2	8 (32%)		
Starch	70	15	60 (86%)	2	8 (12%)		
Low-Fat Protein	55			7	28 (51%)	3	27 (49%)
Medium-Fat Protein	75			7	28 (37%)	5	45 (60%)
High-Fat Protein	95			7	28 (29%)	7	63 (66%)
Fat	45					5	45(100%)
Non-Fat Milk	80	12	48 (60%)	8	32 (40%)	Tr.	
Low-Fat Milk	125	12	48 (38%)	8	32 (27%)	5	45 (36%)
Whole Milk	170	12	48 (28%)	8	32 (19%)	10	90 (53%)

CALCULATING CALORIES

When creating recipes of your own or figuring the portion (exchange) information and calories in other recipes, you will frequently have to work in fractions of portions. I find it is much easier to use a chart giving the exact number of calories available in fractions of portions rather than trying to remember all of the numbers or stopping to re-calculate each time the information is needed. When computing portions and calories for recipes, I always use the same fractions— 1/4,1/2, 3/4—of the whole amount. If the numbers are not exact, I round them off to the nearest fraction. If the amount is well under 1/4 of a whole portion, I drop it completely; however, I am including a 1/8 fraction for the milk group because it allows you much more variety in using your allowed Milk Portions and at the same time monitoring them accurately.

     This is an exact copy of the chart I keep in my own kitchen. I suggest you copy it and put it up in your kitchen:

CALORIES

PORTION*	Whole	Three-Fourths	One-Half	One-Fourth	One-Eighth
Fruit	40	30	20	10	
Vegetable	25	19	13	7	
Starch	70	53	35	18	
Low-Fat Protein	55	42	28	14	
Medium-Fat Protein	75	57	38	19	
High-Fat Protein	95	72	48	24	
Fat	45	34	23	12	
Non-Fat Milk	80	60	40	20	10
Low-Fat Milk	125	94	63	32	16
Whole Milk	170	128	85	43	22

*See the following Food Lists for portion sizes

FRUIT PORTION LIST

Each portion below equals one Fruit Portion and contains
approximately:

10 grams of carbohydrate
40 calories

gm. fiber	mg. chol.	mg. sodium	
1.0	0	1	Apple: 1, 2 inches in diameter
.1	0	.7	Apple juice: 1/3 cup
.6	0	2	Applesauce, unsweetened: 1/2 cup
.6	0	1	Apricots, fresh: 2 medium (Good source of Vitamin A)
.5	0	3	Apricots, dried: 3 halves (Good source of Vitamin A)
			Avocado: see Fat Portion List
.3	0	.5	Banana: 1/2 small
2.0	0	1	Blackberries: 1/2 cup
1.1		1	Blueberries: 1/2 cup
.3	0	10	Cantaloupe: 1/4, 6 inches in diameter (Good source of Vitamins A & C)
.3	0	1	Cherries, sweet: 10 large
1.4	0	2	Cranberries, unsweetened: 1 cup
.3	0	12	Crenshaw melon: 2-inch wedge
.5	0	2	Dates: 2
.5	0	2	Date "sugar": 1 tablespoon
.6	0	1	Figs, fresh: 1 large
.8	0	7	Figs, dried: 1 large
0	0	0	Fructose: 1 tablespoon
.2	0	1	Grapefruit: 1/2, 4 inches in diameter (Good source of Vitamin C)
Tr.	0	1	Grapefruit juice: 1/2 cup (Good source of Vitamin C)
.4	0	2	Grapes: 12 large
.2	0	2	Grapes, Thompson seedless: 20 grapes
Tr.	0	1	Grape juice: 1/4 cup
4.4	0	2	Guava: 2/3 (Good source of Vitamin C)
0	0	1	Honey: 2 teaspoons
.7	0	27	Honeydew melon: 1/4, 5 inches in diameter
.4	0	3	Kiwi: 1 medium
3.0	0	6	Kumquats: 2

gm. fiber	mg. chol.	mg. sodium	
Tr.	0	1	Lemon juice: 1/2 cup
Tr.	0	1	Lime juice: 1/2 cup
.5	0	3.5	Loquats: 3
.2	0	3	Litchi nuts, fresh: 3
.9	0	3	Mango: 1/2 small (Good source of Vitamin A)
0	0	18	Molasses, blackstrap: 1 tablespoon
.3	0	8	Nectarine: 1 medium
.5	0	1	Orange: 1 small (Good source of Vitamin C)
.1	0	1	Orange juice: 1/2 cup (Good source of Vitamin C)
1.0	0	3	Papaya: 1/3 medium (Good source of Vitamin C)
1.5	0	16	Passionfruit: 1
.1	0	28	Passionfruit juice: 1/3 cup
.6	0	1	Peach: 1 medium
1.0	0	3	Pear: 1 small
.8	0	3	Persimmon: 1/2 medium
.3	0	1	Pineapple, fresh or canned without sugar: 1/2 cup
Tr.	0	1	Pineapple juice: 1/3 cup
.2	0	6	Plantain: 1/2 small
.3	0	2	Plums: 2 medium
.2	0	3	Pomegranate: 1 small
.3	0	2	Prunes, fresh or dried: 2
Tr.	0	5	Prune juice: 1/4 cup
.2	0	6	Raisins: 2 tablespoons
3.0	0	1	Raspberries: 1/2 cup
1.5	0	1	Strawberries: 3/4 cup
0	0	0	Sucrose: 1 tablespoon
.5	0	2	Tangerines: 1 large or 2 small
.5	0	1.5	Watermelon: 3/4 cup

VEGETABLE PORTION LIST

Each portion below equals one Vegetable Portion, is equal to one cup
unless otherwise specified, and contains approximately:
5 grams of carbohydrate
2 grams of protein
25 calories
+ Calories negligible when eaten raw
+ + Figures not available

gm. fiber	mg. chol.	mg. sodium	
.6	0	Tr.	Alfalfa sprouts +
4.8	0	40	Artichoke, whole, base and ends of leaves (1 small)
1.0	0	1	Asparagus +
.9	0	5	Bamboo shoots, canned: 3/4 cup
.7	0	4	Bean sprouts +
.8	0	40	Beets (1/2 cup)
1.3	0	37	Beet greens
.6	0	23	Bok choy (Chinese cabbage), raw: 2-1/4 cup
+ +	0	8	Breadfruit (1/4 cup)
1.5	0	22	Broccoli + (Good source of Vitamins A & C)
1.6	0	16	Brussels sprouts (Good source of Vitamin C)
.8	0	16	Cabbage + (Good source of Vitamin C)
1.0	0	24	Carrots (medium) + (Good source of Vitamin A)
1.0	0	12	Cauliflower +
.6	0	100	Celery +
.7	0	100	Celery root (1/2 cup)
.9	0	166	Chard +
.8	0	12	Chayote
.9	0	2	Chicory + (Good source of Vitamin A)
2.0	0	42	Chilies +
1.2	0	16	Chives + (Good source of Vitamins A & C)
.9	0	56	Collards + (Good source of Vitamin C)
1.4	0	24	Coriander (Cilantro) + (1/4 cup)
.6	0	8	Cucumber +
1.6	0	80	Dandelion greens +
1.8	0	2	Eggplant

gm. fiber	mg. chol.	mg. sodium	
1.2	0	10	Endive +
1.0	0	10	Escarole + (Good source of Vitamin A)
.4	0	10	Garlic (1/4 cup)
.5	0	3	Green beans: see String beans
1.0	0	8	Green onion tops +
.3	0	31	Horseradish, prepared (1 tablespoon)
.5	0	30	Jerusalem artichokes (1/2 cup)
.6	0	0.5	Jicama
1.2	0	48	Kale + (Good source of Vitamin C)
.7	0	12	Leeks (1/2 cup)
1.2	0	48	Kale + (Good source of Vitamin C)
.7	0	12	Leeks (1/2 cup)
.6	0	7	Lettuce +
1.8	0	.5	Lima beans, baby (1/4 cup)
.3	0	Tr.	Mint +
.8	0	10	Mushrooms +
.9	0	12	Mustard, fresh + (Good source of Vitamin C)
1.0	0	4	Okra
.6	0	9	Onions (1/2 cup)
1.2	0	30	Palm heart
1.5	0	32	Parsley + (Good source of Vitamins A & C)
.75	0	.4	Peas (1/4 cup)
1.0	0	Tr.	Pea pods, Chinese (1/2 cup)
1.5	0	20	Peppers, green and red + (Good source of Vitamin C)
.6	0	8	Pimiento (1/2 cup)
.9	0	+ +	Poke +
1.3	0	2	Pumpkin (1/2 cup) (Good source of Vitamin C)
.7	0	20	Radishes +
.9	0	2	Rhubarb +
.7	0	4	Romaine lettuce +
1.1	0	4	Rutabagas (1/2 cup)
.8	0	9	Shallots (1/2 cup)
.9	0	37	Spinach +
1.2	0	1	Squash, acorn (1/2 cup)
.2	0	1	Squash, Hubbard (1/2 cup)
3.6	0	2	Squash, spaghetti
1.2	0	6	String beans

gm. fiber	mg. chol.	mg. sodium	
1.2	0	2	Summer squash +
.9	0	6	Tomatoes (1 medium)
.4	0	163	Tomatoes, canned in juice (1/2 cup)
.4	0	6	Tomatoes, canned in juice, unsalted (1/2 cup)
.1	0	282	Tomato catsup, regular (1-1/2 tablespoons)
.1	0	6	Tomato catsup, dietetic, low sodium (1-1/2 tablespoons)
.4	0	244	Tomato juice (1/2 cup)
.4	0	26	Tomato juice, unsalted (1/2 cup)
.3	0	186	Tomato paste (2 tablespoons)
.5	0	12	Tomato paste, unsalted (3 tablespoons)
.6	0	831	Tomato sauce (1/2 cup)
.6	0	42	Tomato sauce, unsalted (1/2 cup)
.8	0	27	Turnips (1/2 cup)
.3	0	550	V-8 juice (2/3 cup) (Good source of Vitamin A)
.3	0	49	V-8 juice, unsalted (2/3 cup) (Good source of Vitamin A)
.2	0	8	Water chestnuts (medium) (4)
.7	0	16	Watercress + (Good source of Vitamin A)
1.4	0	1	Zucchini squash +

STARCH (COMPLEX CARBOHYDRATES) PORTION LIST

Each portion below equals one Starch Portion and contains approximately:

> 15 grams of carbohydrate
> 2 grams of protein
> 70 calories
> + + figures not available

gm. fiber	mg. chol.	mg. sodium	
			STARCHY VEGETABLES AND LEGUMES
1.5	0	3	Beans, dried, cooked, unsalted (lima, soya, navy, pinto, kidney): 1/2 cup
.5	0	1.5	Beans, baked, without salt or pork: 1/4 cup
.6	0	1	Corn, on the cob: 1, 4 inches long
.6	0	1	Corn, cooked and drained: 1/3 cup

gm. fiber	mg. chol.	mg. sodium	
.1	0	Tr.	Hominy, unsalted: 1/2 cup (251 mg. sodium if following directions)
.7	0	14	Lentils, dried, cooked: 1/2 cup
2.0	0	8	Parsnips: 1 small
.5	0	13	Peas, dried, cooked (black-eyed, split): 1/2 cup
.7	0	7	Potatoes, sweet, yams: 1/4 cup (Good source of Vitamin A)
.5	0	2	Potatoes, white, baked or boiled: 1, 2 inches in diameter
.5	0	2	Potatoes, white, mashed: 1/2 cup
.2	0	300	Potato chips: 15, 2 inches in diameter
2.6	0	4	Pumpkin, canned: 1 cup
.2	0	564	Tomato catsup, commercial: 3 tablespoons
.2	0	12	Tomato catsup, dietetic, low sodium, 3 tablespoons
			BREADS
Tr.	0	200	Bagel: 1/2
Tr.	0	185	Biscuit: 1, 2 inches in diameter
.1	0	7	Bread, low sodium: 1 slice
.1	0	139	Bread, rye: 1 slice
.4	0	136	Bread, whole wheat: 1 slice
Tr.	0	148	Bread (white and sourdough): 1 slice
Tr.	0	200	Breadsticks: 4, 7 inches long
Tr.	0	116	Bun, hamburger: 1/2
Tr.	0	153	Bun, hot dog: 2/3
.4	0	130	Chapati, whole wheat: 1, 6 inches in diameter
.1	0	245	Corn bread: 1 piece 1-1/2 inches square
Tr.	0	140	Croutons, plain: 1/2 cup
.1	0	7	Croutons, plain, low-sodium bread: 1/2 cup
Tr.	0	133	English muffin: 1/2
Tr.	0	1	Matzo cracker, plain: 1, 6 inches in diameter
Tr.	0	222	Melba Toast: 6 slices
Tr.	0	117	Muffin, unsweetened: 1, 2 inches in diameter
Tr.	0	412	Pancakes: 2, 3 inches in diameter
Tr.	0	7	Pancakes, low sodium: 2, 3 inches in diameter
Tr.	0	128	Pita bread: 1/2 of 6-inch pocket
Tr.	0	88	Popover: 1
+ +	0	1.3	Rice cakes, unsalted: 2
Tr.	0	143	Roll: 1, 2 inches in diameter
Tr.	0	70	Rusks: 2

gm. fiber	mg. chol.	mg. sodium	
.1	0	712	Spoon bread: 1/2 cup
.3	0	Tr.	Tortilla, corn, flour: 1, 7 inches in diameter
Tr.	0	203	Waffle: 1, 4 inches in diameter
			CEREALS
2.4	0	287	All-Bran: 1/2 cup
2.0	0	94	Bran Flakes: 1/2 cup
.2	0	240	Cheerios: 1 cup
.2	0	72	Concentrate: 1/4 cup
.1	0	178	Corn Flakes: 2/3 cup
Tr.	0	7	Cream of Rice, cooked: 1/2 cup
Tr.	0	1	Cream of Wheat, cooked: 1/2 cup
.4	0	147	Grapenuts: 1/4 cup
.3	0	113	Grapenut Flakes: 1/2 cup
.1	0	1	Grits, cooked: 1/2 cup
Tr.	0	165	Kix: 3/4 cup
.3	0	132	Life: 1/2 cup
Tr.	0	1	Malt-O-Meal, cooked: 1/2 cup
Tr.	0	2	Maypo, cooked: 1/2 cup
Tr.	0	1	Matzo meal, cooked: 1/2 cup
2.0	0	195	Nutri-Grain: 1/2 cup
.2	0	1	Oatmeal, cooked: 1/2 cup
.2	0	92	Pep: 1/2 cup
.2	0	1	Puffed rice: 1-1/2 cups
.3	0	1	Puffed wheat: 1-1/2 cups
Tr.	0	174	Rice Krispies: 2/3 cup
.4	0	Tr.	Roman Meal, cooked: 1/2 cup
1.0	0	.5	Rye cereal, cooked: 1/2 cup
.4	0	1	Shredded wheat biscuit: 1 large
.3	0	168	Special K: 1-1/4 cups
.4	0	163	Wheat Chex: 1/2 cup
.4	0	Tr.	Wheatena, cooked: 1/2 cup
.2	0	210	Wheaties: 2/3 cup
			GRAINS
.1	0	Tr.	Barley, cooked: 1/2 cup
3.3	0	Tr.	Bran, unprocessed rice: 1/3 cup
3.2	0	Tr.	Bran, unprocessed wheat: 1/3 cup
.3	0	4	Buckwheat groats (kasha), cooked: 1/3 cup

gm. fiber	mg. chol.	mg. sodium	
.3	0	4	Bulgur (cracked wheat), cooked: 1/2 cup
1.5	0	.25	Corn germ: 2 tablespoons
.1	0	1	Cornmeal, cooked: 1/2 cup
.3	0	4	Cracked wheat (bulgur), cooked: 1/2 cup
.3	0	4	Kasha (buckwheat groats), cooked: 1/3 cup
1.6	0	.5	Millet, cooked: 1/2 cup
.3	0	.5	Oatmeal, uncooked: 1/4 cup
.3	0	1	Popcorn, popped, unbuttered & unsalted: 3 cups
.2	0	6	Rice, brown, cooked, unsalted: 1/3 cup
Tr.	0	3	Rice, white, cooked, unsalted: 1/2 cup
.3	0	4	Rice, wild, cooked, unsalted: 1/2 cup
+ +	0	.5	Soya granules: 2 tablespoons
.2	0	1	Steel cut oats, cooked: 1/2 cup
Tr.	0	1	Wheat germ, defatted: 1 ounce or 3 tablespoons
			FLOURS
Tr.	0	2	Arrowroot: 2 tablespoons
Tr.	0	1	All purpose: 2-1/2 tablespoons
Tr.	0	138	Bisquick: 1-1/2 tablespoons
3.2	0	Tr.	Bran, unprocessed wheat: 5 tablespoons
.3	0	1	Buckwheat: 3 tablespoons
Tr.	0	1	Cake: 2-1/2 tablespoons
.1	0	Tr.	Cornmeal: 3 tablespoons
Tr.	0	Tr.	Cornstarch: 2 tablespoons
Tr.	0	1	Matzo meal: 3 tablespoons
Tr.	0	12	Potato flour: 2-1/2 tablespoons
.4	0	4	Rice flour: 3 tablespoons
.5	0	1	Rye, dark: 4 tablespoons
Tr.	0	1.5	Soya powder: 3 tablespoons
.6	0	1	Whole wheat: 3 tablespoons
			PASTAS
Tr.	0	1	Noodles, macaroni, spaghetti, cooked: 1/2 cup
Tr.	9.4	2	Noodles, dry, egg: 3-1/2 ounces
Tr.	3.1	1.5	Noodles, cooked, egg: 3-1/2 ounces
Tr.	0	.5	Noodles, rice, cooked: 1/2 cup
.4	0	1.5	Noodles, whole wheat, cooked: 1/2 cup
Tr.	0	.5	Pasta, enriched white, cooked: 1/2 cup
.4	0	1.5	Pasta, whole wheat, cooked: 1/2 cup

gm. fiber	mg. chol.	mg. sodium	
			CRACKERS
Tr.	0	48	Animal: 8
Tr.	0	33	Arrowroot: 3
Tr.	0	164	Cheese tidbits: 1/2 cup
.2	0	88	Graham: 2
.2	0	10	Low sodium: 4
Tr.	0	220	Oyster: 20 or 1/2 cup
Tr.	0	90	Pretzels: 10 very thin, or 1 large
Tr.	0	250	Saltines: 5, salted
Tr.	0	69	Soda: 3, unsalted
Tr.	0	192	Ritz: 6
.3	0	225	RyKrisp: 3
.3	0	130	Rye thins: 10
Tr.	0	336	Triangle thins: 14
.4	0	150	Triscuits: 5
Tr.	0	172	Vegetable thins: 12
Tr.	0	276	Wheat thins: 12
			MISCELLANEOUS
1.8	0	10	Cocoa, dry, unsweetened: 2-1/2 tablespoons
.2	0	120	Fritos: 3/4 ounce or 1/2 cup
0	26.3	40	Ice cream, low saturated fat: 1/2 cup

LOW-FAT PROTEIN PORTION LIST

Each portion below equals one Low-Fat Protein Portion and contains approximately:

7 grams of protein
3 grams of fat
55 calories

gm. fiber	mg. chol.	mg. sodium	
			CHEESE
0	2.6	234	Cottage cheese, low-fat: 1/4 cup
0	1.3	90	Cottage cheese, dry curd: 1/4 cup
0	3.0	222	Farmers': 1/4 cup, crumbled, salted
0	3.0	75	Farmers': 1/4 cup crumbled, unsalted

gm. fiber	mg. chol.	mg. sodium	
0	3.0	+ +	Hoop (Bakers'): 1/4 cup
0	3.0	12	Pot: 1/4 cup
0	18.2	46	Ricotta, part skim: 1/4 cup or 2 ounces
			EGG WHITE AND EGG SUBSTITUTES
0	0	47	Egg white: 1 (4 gr. protein)
0	0	130	Liquid egg substitute: 1/4 cup (sodium content varies with brands)
0	0	132	Dry egg substitute: 3 tablespoons
			CHICKEN
0	25.8	22	Broiled or roasted: 1 ounce or 1 slice $3 \times 2 \times 1/8$ inch
0	22.4	19	Breast, without skin: 1/2 small, 1 ounce or 1/4 cup, chopped
0	25.8	25	Leg: 1/2 medium or 1 ounce
			TURKEY
0	22.4	23	Meat, white, without skin: 1 ounce or 1 slice $3 \times 2 \times 1/8$ inch
0	25.8	28	Meat, dark, without skin: 1 ounce or 1 slice $3 \times 2 \times 1/8$ inch
			OTHER POULTRY AND GAME
0	30.0	25	Buffalo: 1 ounce or 1 slice $3 \times 2 \times 1/8$ inch
0	22.4	22	Cornish game hen, without skin: 1/4 bird or 1 ounce
0	21.4	20	Pheasant: 1-1/2 ounces
0	25.8	18	Rabbit: 1 ounce or 1 slice $3 \times 2 \times 1/8$ inch
0	21.4	12	Quail, without skin: 1/4 bird or 1 ounce
0	21.4	22	Squab, without skin: 1/4 bird or 1 ounce
0	25.7	25	Venison, lean, roast or steak: 1 ounce or 1 slice $3 \times 2 \times 1/8$ inch
			FISH AND SHELLFISH
0	24.4	95	Abalone: 1-1/3 ounces
0	18.3	112	Albacore, canned in oil: 1 ounce
0	21.4	2640	Anchovy fillets: 9
0	12.5	1540	Anchovy paste: 1 tablespoon
0	27.1	15	Bass: 1-1/2 ounces
0	85.7	624	Caviar: 1 ounce
0	Tr.	612	Clam juice: 1-1/2 cups
0	18.0	51	Clams, fresh: 3 large or 1-1/2 ounces
0	27.0	190	Clams, canned: 1-1/2 ounces
0	18.1	31	Cod: 1 ounce
0	43.0	77	Crab, canned: 1/2 ounce

gm. fiber	mg. chol.	mg. sodium	
0	42.5	90	Crab, cracked, fresh: 1-1/2 ounces
0	30.2	110	Flounder: 1-2/3 ounces
0	55.0	84	Frog legs: 2 large or 3 ounces
0	18.1	30	Halibut: 1 ounce or 1 piece 2 × 2 × 1 inch
0	27.0	2000	Herring, pickled: 1-1/4 ounces
0	94.0	2207	Herring, smoked: 1-1/4 ounces
0	31.0	90	Lobster, fresh, 1-1/2 ounces, 1/4 cup or 1/4 small lobster
0	36.0	90	Lobster, canned, unsalted: 1-1/2 ounces
0	23.0	31	Oysters, fresh: 3 medium or 1-1/2 ounces
0	25.5	171	Oysters, canned, 1-1/2 ounces
0	27.1	39	Perch: 1-1/2 ounces
0	27.1	38	Red snapper: 1-1/2 ounces
0	18.4	14	Salmon: 1 ounce
0	16.0	235	Salmon, canned: 1-1/2 ounces
0	18.0	261	Salmon, smoked (lox): 1-1/2 ounces
0	24.4	33	Sanddabs: 1-1/2 ounces
0	40.0	108	Sardines: 4 small
0	40.0	26	Sardines, unsalted: 4 small
0	23.0	112	Scallops: 3 medium or 1-1/2 ounces
0	48.0	60	Shrimp, fresh: 5 medium
0	64.0	420	Shrimp, canned: 5 medium or 1-1/2 ounces
0	30.0	44	Sole: 1-2/3 ounces
0	27.1	40	Swordfish: 1-1/2 ounces
0	27.1	11	Trout: 1-1/2 ounces
0	18.1	10	Tuna, fresh: 1 ounce
0	25.2	370	Tuna, canned in oil: 1/4 cup
0	25.2	25	Tuna, unsalted, water packed (dietetic): 1/4 cup
0	27.1	32	Turbot: 1-1/2 ounces
			BEEF
0	41.8	26	Flank steak: 1-1/2 ounces
0	31.3	17	Rib roast: 1 ounce, 1/4 cup, chopped, or 1 slice 3 × 2 × 1/8 inch
0	30.0	17	Steak, very lean (filet mignon, New York, sirloin, T-bone): 1 ounce or 1 slice 3 × 2 × 1/8 inch
0	Tr.	21	Tripe: 1 ounce or 1 piece 5 × 2 inches
			LAMB
0	28.0	20	Chops, lean: 1/2 small chop or 1 ounce

gm. fiber	mg. chol.	mg. sodium	
0	27.7	20	Roast, lean: 1 ounce, 1 slice 3 × 2 × 1/8 inch, or 1/4 cup, chopped
			PORK
0	25.3	264	Ham: 1 ounce or 1 slice 3 × 2 × 1/8 inch
			VEAL
0	28.7	23	Chop: 1/2 small or 1 ounce
0	29.0	23	Cutlet: 1 ounce or 1 slice 3 × 2 × 1/8 inch
0	28.7	23	Roast: 1 ounce or 1 slice 3 × 2 × 1/8 inch

MEDIUM-FAT PROTEIN PORTION LIST

Each portion below equals one Medium-Fat Protein Portion and contains approximately:

7 grams of protein

5 grams of fat

75 calories

gm. fiber	mg. chol.	mg. sodium	
			CHEESE
0	8.4	130	Cottage cheese, creamed: 1/4 cup
0	16.0	312	Feta: 1 ounce
0	17.4	227	Mozzarella: 1 ounce
0	14.8	163	Parmesan: 1/4 cup, 2/3 ounce or 4 tablespoons
0	29.1	46	Ricotta: regular: 1/4 cup or 2 ounces
0	14.8	247	Romano: 1/4 cup, 2/3 ounce or 4 tablespoons
			EGGS
0	250.0	59	Egg, medium: 1
			Egg white (see Low-Fat Protein)
0	250.0	12	Egg yolk: 1 (3 gr. protein; 5 grams fat)
			CHICKEN
0	55	16	Gizzard: 1 ounce
0	66	20	Heart: 1 ounce
0	211.4	17	Liver: 1 ounce
			BEEF
0	571.4	54	Brains: 1 ounce

gm. fiber	mg. chol.	mg. sodium	
0	26.0	298	Corned beef, canned: 1 ounce or 1 slice 3 × 2 × 1/8 inch
0	30.3	14	Hamburger, very lean (4 ounces raw = 3 ounces cooked): 1 ounce
0	42.8	30	Heart: 1 ounce or 1 slice 3 × 2 × 1/8 inch
0	107.1	72	Kidney: 1 ounce or 1 slice 3 × 2 × 1/8 inch
0	124.1	59	Liver: 1 ounce or 1 slice 3 × 2 × 1/8 inch
0	46	17	Tongue: 1 slice 3 × 2 × 1/8 inch
			PORK
0	25.3	343	Canadian bacon: 1 slice 2-1/2 inches in diameter, 1/4 inch thick
0	25.0	18	Chops, lean: 1/2 small chop or 1 ounce
0	42.9	19	Heart: 1 ounce
0	124.1	30	Liver: 1 ounce
0	25.0	18	Roast, lean: 1 ounce, 1 slice 3 × 2 × 1/8 inch or 1/4 cup, chopped
			VEAL
0	124.1	30	Calves' liver: 1 ounce or 1 slice 3 × 2 × 1/8 inch
0	71.4	33	Sweetbreads: 1 ounce, 1/4 pair or 1/4 cup, chopped
0	28.7	22	Roast, lean: 1 ounce, 1/4 cup, chopped, or 1 slice 3 × 2 × 1/8 inch
			VEGETABLES
.1	0	7	Tofu (soybean curd): 4 ounces, 1/2 cup or 1 slice 2 × 2 × 1-1/2 inches

HIGH-FAT PROTEIN PORTION LIST

Each portion below equals one High-Fat Protein Portion and contains approximately:

7 grams of protein
7 grams of fat
95 calories
+ + Figures not available

gm. fiber	mg. chol.	mg. sodium	
			CHEESE
0	28.4	193	American: 1 ounce
0	21.2	510	Bleu: 1 ounce or 1/4 cup, crumbled

gm. fiber	mg. chol.	mg. sodium	
0	30.1	193	Cheddar: 1 ounce
0	30.1	10	Cheddar, low sodium: 1 ounce (sodium content varies with brands)
0	29.1	204	Edam: 1 ounce
0	21.0	271	Liederkranz: 1 ounce
0	18.0	204	Monterey Jack: 1 ounce
0	25.0	204	Muenster: 1 ounce
Tr.	18.2	465	Pimiento cheese spread: 1 ounce
0	24.0	465	Roquefort: 1 ounce or 1/4 cup, crumbed
0	21.0	+ +	Stilton: 1 ounce or 1/4 cup, crumbled
0	28.0	85	Swiss: 1 ounce
			COLD CUTS
0	25.9	266	Bologna: 1 ounce or 1 slice 4-1/2 inches in diameter, 1/8 inch thick
0	35.0	264	Liverwurst: 1 slice 3 inches in diameter, 1/4 inch thick
0	25.9	340	Spam: 1 ounce
0	25.9	425	Salami: 1 ounce or 1 slice 4-1/2 inches in diameter, 1/8 inch thick
0	25.9	228	Vienna sausage: 2-1/2 sausages or 1 ounce
			DUCK
0	16.0	21	Roasted, without skin: 1 ounce or 1 slice 3 × 2 × 1/8 inch
0	16.0	28	Wild duck, without skin: 1 ounce
			BEEF
0	31.3	17	Brisket: 1 ounce
0	25.9	508	Frankfurters: 1 (8 to 9 per pound)
0	31.3	18	Short ribs, very lean: 1 rib or 1 ounce
			PEANUT BUTTER
.3	0	156	Peanut butter, regular: 2 tablespoons
.3	0	6	Peanut butter, unsalted: 2 tablespoons
			PORK
			Bacon (see Fat Portion List)
0	25.9	250	Sausage: 2 small or 1 ounce
0	25.3	19	Spareribs, without fat: meat from 3 medium or 1 ounce

FAT PORTION LIST

Each portion below equals one Fat Portion and contains approximately:

5 grams of fat
45 calories
+ + Figures not available

gm. fiber	mg. chol.	mg. sodium	
.8	0	1	Avocado: 1/8, 4 inches in diameter
0	7.0	209	Bacon, crisp: 1 slice
0	12.0	39	Butter: 1 teaspoon
0	13.0	.3	Butter, unsalted: 1 teaspoon
1.2	0	5	Caraway seeds: 2 tablespoons
1.2	0	5	Cardamom seeds: 2 tablespoons
0	0	4	Chocolate, bitter: 1/3 ounce or 1/3 square
0	10.0	35	Cream cheese: 1 tablespoon
0	20.0	5	Cream, heavy, whipping: 1 tablespoon
0	20.0	12	Cream, light, coffee: 2 tablespoons
0	17.0	18	Cream, half-and-half: 3 tablespoons
0	16.0	12	Cream, sour: 2 tablespoons
0	0	32	Cream, sour, imitation: 2 tablespoons (Imo, Matey)
0	0	35	Margarine, polyunsaturated: 1 teaspoon
0	0	.8	Margarine, polyunsaturated, unsalted: 1 teaspoon
0	2.6	25	Mayonnaise: 1 teaspoon
0	0	0	Oils: 1 teaspoon
.6	0	384	Olives, green: 4 medium
.6	0	125	Olives, ripe: 5 small
.8	0	3	Poppy seeds: 1-1/2 tablespoons
.2	0	Tr.	Pumpkin seeds: 1-1/2 teaspoons
.2	0	4	Sesame seeds: 2 teaspoons
.2	0	3	Sunflower seeds: 1-1/2 teaspoons
			SALAD DRESSINGS, COMMERCIAL
Tr.	1.3	59	Bleu cheese: 1 teaspoon
Tr.	0.3	95	Bleu cheese, diet, sugar: 1 teaspoon
Tr.	0	57	Caesar: 1 teaspoon
Tr.	0	77	French: 1 teaspoon

gm. fiber	mg. chol.	mg. sodium	
Tr.	0	74	Italian: 1 teaspoon
Tr.	0	64	Italian, diet: 1 teaspoon
Tr.	1.3	48	Roquefort: 1 teaspoon
Tr.	3.0	44	Thousand Island, diet: 1 teaspoon
Tr.	.3	33	Thousand Island, egg-free: 1 teaspoon
			SAUCES, COMMERCIAL:
Tr.	.6	60	Bearnaise: 1 teaspoon
Tr.	8.0	28	Hollandaise: 1 teaspoon
Tr.	1.3	61	Tartar: 1 teaspoon
			NUTS, UNSALTED
.3	0	.5	Almonds: 7
.2	0	.5	Brazil nuts: 2
.2	0	2	Cashews: 7
.5	0	5	Coconut, fresh: 1 piece 1 × 1 × 3/8 inch
.3	0	5	Coconut, shredded, unsweetened: 2 tablespoons
1.2	0	.5	Filberts: 5
1.2	0	.5	Hazelnuts: 5
.1	0	Tr.	Hickory nuts: 7 small
.3	0	1	Macadamia nuts: 2
.4	0	1	Peanuts, Spanish: 20
.4	0	1	Peanuts, Virginia: 10
.3	0	Tr.	Pecans: 6 halves
.2	0	Tr.	Pine nuts: 1 tablespoon
.1	0	Tr.	Pistachio nuts: 15
.2	0	19	Soy nuts, toasted: 3 tablespoons
.2	0	.5	Walnuts, black: 5 halves
.2	0	.5	Walnuts, California: 5 halves

NON-FAT MILK PORTION LIST

Each portion below equals one Non-Fat Milk Portion and contains approximately:

12 grams of carbohydrate
8 grams of protein
Trace of fat
80 calories
+ + Figures not available

gm. fiber	mg. chol.	mg. sodium	
0	7.8	280	Buttermilk: 1 cup
0	2.0	155	Milk, powdered, skim, dry: 3 tablespoons
0	1.7	115	Milk, powdered, skim, mixed: 1/4 cup
0	5.0	127	Milk, skim, non-fat: 1 cup
0	11.0	121	Milk, skim, instant: 1 cup
0	2.3	165	Milk, evaporated, skim: 1/2 cup
0	13.0	75	Sherbet: 1 cup
Tr.	0	2	Soya powder (Fearn): 3 tablespoons
0	14.0	116	Yogurt, plain, non-fat: 1 cup

LOW-FAT MILK PORTION LIST

Each portion below equals one Low-Fat Milk Portion and contains approximately:

12 grams of carbohydrate
8 grams of protein
5 grams of fat
125 calories

gm. fiber	mg. chol.	mg. sodium	
0	14.0	115	Kefir, Plain, low-fat: 1 cup
0	15.5	150	Milk, low-fat, 2% fat: 1 cup
0	15.0	12	Milk, low sodium, canned (LSM): 1 cup
0	17.0	115	Yogurt, plain, low-fat: 1 cup

WHOLE MILK PORTION LIST

Each portion below equals one Whole Milk Portion and contains approximately:

12 grams of carbohydrate
8 grams of protein
10 grams of fat
170 calories
+ + Figures not available

gm. fiber	mg. chol.	mg. sodium	
0	26.0	136	Ice milk: 1 cup
0	30.0	114	Kefir, plain, whole: 1 cup
0	32.7	120	Milk, whole: 1 cup
0	32.7	149	Milk, evaporated, whole: 1/2 cup
0	30.0	114	Yogurt, plain, whole: 1 cup

HERBS, SPICES, SEASONINGS, ETC.

Calories are negligible and need not be counted in the following list; however, many of these foods are extremely high in sodium and must be calculated very carefully.

gm. fiber	mg. chol.	mg. sodium	
0	0	250	Baking powder: 1 teaspoon
0	0	Tr.	Baking powder, low sodium: 1 teaspoon
0	0	1360	Baking soda: 1 teaspoon
Tr.	0	10	Bakon Seasoning: 1 teaspoon (12 calories)
0	0	Tr.	Bitters, Angostura: 1 teaspoon
0	0	425	Bouillon cube, beef (fat free): 1-1/2-inch cube or 4 grams
0	0	10	Bouillon cube, beef (fat free and salt free): 1-1/2-inch cube or 4 grams
0	0	5	Bouillon cube, chicken (fat free and salt free): 1-1/2-inch cube or 4 grams
Tr.	0	3006	Capers: 1 tablespoon
0	2.0	737	Chicken stock, commercial: 1 cup

gm. fiber	mg. chol.	mg. sodium	
0	2.0	200	Chicken stock, homemade: 1 cup
.9	0	294	Chutney: 1 tablespoon (Crosse & Blackwell's; Major Grey's)
0	0	1	Coffee: 1 cup
0	0	Tr.	Extracts: 1 teaspoon
0	0	4	Gelatin, unsweetened: 1 envelope (1 scant tablespoon)
0	0	55	Kitchen bouquet: 1 tablespoon
0	0	0	Liquid smoke: 1 teaspoon
Tr.	0	63	Mustard, prepared: 1 teaspoon (French's)
Tr.	0	34	Mustard, prepared low sodium: 1 teaspoon
Tr.	0	1.3	Mustard, Dijon style, low sodium: 1 teaspoon
Tr.	0	811	Pickles: 1 2-ounce, without sugar
0	0	6	Rennet tablets: 1 ounce
0	0	1938	Salt: 1 teaspoon
0	0	2077	Soy sauce: 1 ounce (2 tablespoons)
0	0	1210	Soy sauce, salt reduced: 2 tablespoons
0	0	6	Tabasco sauce: 1/4 teaspoon
0	0	Tr.	Vinegar, cider: 1 tablespoon
0	0	5	Vinegar, red wine: 1 tablespoon
0	0	5	Vinegar, rice: 1 tablespoon
0	0	5	Vinegar, white wine: 1 tablespoon
0	0	58	Worcestershire sauce: 1 tablespoon (Lea & Perrins)
.4	0	2	Allspice, ground: 1 teaspoon
.4	0	1	Allspice, whole: 1 teaspoon
.3	0	Tr.	Aniseed: 1 teaspoon
.2	0	Tr.	Basil: 1 teaspoon
.3	0	Tr.	Bay leaf: 1 leaf
.2	0	4	Celery seed, ground: 1 teaspoon
.2	0	2	Celery seed, whole: 1 teaspoon
.3	0	31	Chili powder, seasoned: 1 teaspoon
.3	0	Tr.	Cinnamon, ground: 1 teaspoon
.2	0	3	Cloves, ground: 1 teaspoon
.2	0	1	Cloves, whole: 1 teaspoon
.4	0	Tr.	Coriander, ground: 1 teaspoon
.1	0	Tr.	Cumin seed: 1 teaspoon
.3	0	1	Curry powder: 1 teaspoon
.4	0	Tr.	Dill seed: 1 teaspoon
.1	0	Tr.	Dill weed: 1 teaspoon

gm. fiber	mg. chol.	mg. sodium	
.4	0	1	Fennel seed: 1 teaspoon
Tr.	0	1	Garlic powder: 1 teaspoon
.1	0	1	Ginger, ground: 1 teaspoon
.3	0	Tr.	Juniper berries: 1 teaspoon
Tr.	0	Tr.	Lemon peel, dried: 1 teaspoon
Tr.	0	Tr.	Lemon peel, fresh: 1 teaspoon
Tr.	0	2	Mace, ground: 1 teaspoon
Tr.	0	Tr.	Marjoram, dried: 1 teaspoon
Tr.	0	Tr.	Mint, dried: 1 teaspoon
.4	0	Tr.	Mustard seed: 1 teaspoon
Tr.	0	Tr.	Nutmeg, ground: 1 teaspoon
.1	0	2	Onion powder: 1 teaspoon
.3	0	Tr.	Oregano, dried: 1 teaspoon
.4	0	1	Paprika, ground: 1 teaspoon
.1	0	5	Parsley flakes: 1 teaspoon
.2	0	Tr.	Pepper, black: 1 teaspoon
.5	0	Tr.	Pepper, cayenne: 1 teaspoon
.3	0	698	Pepper, lemon: 1 teaspoon (Durkee's)
.1	0	Tr.	Pepper, white: 1 teaspoon
.2	0	Tr.	Rosemary, dried: 1 teaspoon
Tr.	0	Tr.	Saffron, powdered: 1 teaspoon
.1	0	Tr.	Sage, dried: 1 teaspoon
.2	0	Tr.	Savory, dried: 1 teaspoon
.1	0	Tr.	Tarragon, dried: 1 teaspoon
.1	0	Tr.	Thyme, dried: 1 teaspoon
.1	0	1	Turmeric, ground: 1 teaspoon

ALCOHOLIC BEVERAGES

Whether you are allowed alcoholic beverages in your diet should be decided between you and your doctor. There is no question that weight loss and weight maintenance are simplified greatly by not drinking, as liquor of all types is high in calories. Also, as you will notice by the figures given, many alcoholic beverages are also high in sodium.

C = calories

GC = grams of carbohydrates

gm. fiber	mg. chol.	mg. sodium	
			BEER AND ALE
0	0	17	Ale, mild, 8 oz. = 98 C, 8 GC
0	0	8	Beer, 8 oz. = 114 C, 11 GC
			WINES
0	0	3	Champagne, brut, 3 oz. = 75 C, 1 GC
0	0	3	Champagne, extra dry, 3 oz. = 87 C, 4 GC
0	0	4	Dubonnet, 3 oz. = 96 C, 7 GC
0	0	4	Dry Marsala, 3 oz. = 162 C, 18 GC
0	0	4	Sweet Marsala, 3 oz. = 152 C, 23 GC
0	0	4	Muscatel, 4 oz. = 158 C, 14 GC
0	0	4	Port, 4 oz. = 158 C, 14 GC
0	0	4	Red wine, dry, 3 oz. = 69 C, under 1 GC
0	0	4	Sake, 3 oz. = 75 C, 6 GC
0	0	4	Sherry, domestic, 3-1/2 oz. = 84 C, 5 GC
0	0	4	Dry vermouth, 3-1/2 oz. = 105 C, 1 GC
0	0	4	Sweet vermouth, 3-1/2 oz. = 167 C, 12 GC
0	0	4	White wine, dry, 3 oz. = 74 C, under 1 GC
			LIQUEURS AND CORDIALS
0	0	2	Amaretto, 1 oz. = 112 C, 13 GC
0	0	2	Crème de Cacao, 1 oz. = 101 C, 12 GC
0	0	2	Crème de Menthe, 1 oz. = 112 C, 13 GC
0	0	2	Curaçao, 1 oz. = 100 C, 9 GC
0	0	2	Drambuie, 1 oz. = 110 C, 11 GC
0	0	2	Tia Maria, 1 oz. = 113 C, 9 GC
			SPIRITS
			Bourbon, brandy, Cognac, Canadian whiskey, gin,rye, rum, scotch, tequila and vodka are all carbohydrate free! The calories they contain depend upon the proof.
0	0	Tr.	80 proof, 1 oz. = 67 C
0	0	Tr.	84 proof, 1 oz. = 70 C
0	0	Tr.	90 proof, 1 oz. = 75 C
0	0	Tr.	94 proof, 1 oz. = 78 C
0	0	Tr.	97 proof, 1 oz. = 81 C
0	0	Tr.	100 proof, 1 oz. = 83 C

TABLE OF EQUIVALENTS

BEVERAGES
ICE CUBES
2 ice cubes = 1/4 cup
8 ice cubes = 1 cup
INSTANT COFFEE
4-ounce jar = 60 cups coffee
COFFEE
1 pound (80 tablespoons) = 40 to 50 cups
TEA LEAVES
1 pound = 300 cups tea

BREADS
CRUMBS
Bread crumbs, soft, 1 slice = 3/4 cup
Bread crumbs, dry, crumbled, 2 slices = 1/2 cup
Bread crumbs, dry, ground, 4 slices = 1/2 cup
Graham crackers, 14 squares, fine crumbs = 1 cup
Soda crackers, 21 squares, fine crumbs = 1 cup
CEREALS AND NOODLES
Flour, cake, 1 pound = 4-1/2 cups, sifted
Flour, all purpose, 1 pound = 4 cups, sifted
Bulgur, 1/3 cup = 1 cup, cooked
Cornmeal, 1 cup = 4 cups, cooked
Macaroni, 1 pound, 5 cups = 12 cups, cooked
Noodles, 1 pound, 5-1/2 cups = 10 cups, cooked
Oatmeal, 1 cup = 2 cups, cooked; 1-1/2 cups ground = 1 cup oat flour
Spaghetti, 1 pound = 9 cups, cooked

FATS
MISCELLANEOUS
Bacon, 1 pound, rendered = 1-1/2 cups
Bacon, 1 slice, cooked crisp = 1 tablespoon, crumbled
Butter, 1 cube (1/4 pound) = 1/2 cup or 8 tablespoons
Cheese, cream, 3-ounce package = 6 tablespoons
Cream, heavy whipping, 1 cup = 2 cups, whipped
Margarine, 1 cube (1/4 pound) = 1/2 cup or 8 tablespoons
NUTS IN THE SHELL
Almonds, 1 pound = 1 cup nutmeats
Brazil nuts, 1 pound = 1-1/2 cups nutmeats
Peanuts, 1 pound = 2 cups nutmeats
Pecans, 1 pound = 2-1/2 cups nutmeats
Walnuts, 1 pound = 2-1/3 cups nutmeats
NUTS, SHELLED
Almonds, 1/2 pound = 2 cups
Almonds, 56, chopped = 1/2 cup
Brazil nuts, 1/2 pound = 1-1/2 cups
Coconut, 1/2 pound, shredded = 2-1/2 cups
Macadamia nuts, 3, finely chopped = 1 tablespoon
Peanuts, 1/2 pound = 1 cup
Peanuts, 50, chopped = 1/2 cup
Pecans, 1/2 pound = 2 cups
Pecans, 42 halves, chopped = 1/2 cup
Walnuts, 1/2 pound = 2 cups
Walnuts, 15 halves, chopped = 1/2 cup

FRUIT (DRIED)
Apricots, 24 halves, 1 cup = 1-1/2 cups, cooked
Dates, 1 pound, 2-1/2 cups = 1-3/4 cups, pitted and chopped; 12 dates, pitted and chopped = 1/2 cup

Figs, 1 pound, 2-1/2 cups = 4-1/2 cups, cooked

Pears, 1 pound, 3 cups = 5-1/2 cups, cooked

Prunes, pitted, 1 pound, 2-1/2 cups = 3-3/4 cups, cooked

Raisins, seedless, 1 pound, 2-3/4 cups = 3-3/4 cups, cooked

FRUIT (FRESH)

Apples, 1 pound, 4 small = 3 cups, chopped

Apricots, 1 pound, 6 to 8 average = 2 cups, chopped

Bananas, 1 pound, 4 small = 2 cups, mashed

Berries, 1 pint = 2 cups

Cantaloupe, 2 pounds, 1 average = 3 cups, diced

Cherries, 1 pint = 1 cup, pitted

Cranberries, 1 pound = 4-1/2 cups

Crenshaw melon, 3 pounds, 1 average = 4-1/2 cups, diced

Figs, 1 pound, 4 small = 2 cups, chopped

Grapefruit, 1 small = 1 cup, sectioned

Grapes, Concord, 1/4 pound, 30 grapes = 1 cup

Grapes, Thompson seedless, 1/4 pound, 40 grapes = 1 cup

Guavas, 1 pound, 4 medium = 1 cup, chopped

Honeydew melon, 2 pounds, 1 average = 3 cups, diced

Kumquats, 1 pound, 8 to 10 average = 2 cups, sliced

Lemon, 1 medium (3 average = 1 pound) = 3 tablespoons juice; 2 teaspoons grated peel

Limes, 1/2 pound, 5 average = 4 tablespoons juice; 4 to 5 tablespoons grated peel

Loquats, 1 pound, 5 average = 1-1/2 cups, chopped

Lychees, 1 pound, 6 average = 1/2 cup, chopped

Mangoes, 1 pound, 2 average = 1-1/2 cups, chopped

Nectarines, 1 pound, 3 average = 2 cups, chopped

Orange, 1 small (2 average = 1 pound) = 6 tablespoons juice; 1 tablespoon grated peel; 3/4 cup, sectioned

Papaya, 1 medium = 1-1/2 cups, chopped

Peaches, 1 pound, 3 average = 2 cups, chopped

Pears, 1 pound, 3 average = 2 cups, chopped

Persimmons, 1 pound, 3 average = 2 cups, mashed

Pineapple, 3 pounds, 1 medium = 2-1/2 cups, chopped

Plums, 1 pound, 4 average = 2 cups, chopped

Pomegranate, 1/4 pound, 1 average = 3 cups seeds

Prunes, 1 pound, 5 average = 2 cups, chopped

Rhubarb, 1 pound, 4 slender stalks = 2 cups, cooked

Tangerines, 1 pound, 4 average = 2 cups, sectioned

Watermelon, 10 to 12 pounds, 1 average = 20 to 24 cups, cubed

HERBS, SPICES AND SEASONINGS

Garlic powder, 1/8 teaspoon = 1 small clove garlic

Ginger, powdered, 1/2 teaspoon = 1 teaspoon, fresh

Herbs, dried, 1/2 teaspoon = 1 tablespoon, fresh

Horseradish, bottled, 2 tablespoons = 1 tablespoon, fresh

MILK

Dry, whole powdered milk, 1/4 cup + 1 cup water = 1 cup whole milk

Dry, instant non-fat powdered milk, 1/3 cup + 2/3 cup water = 1 cup non-fat milk

Dry, non-instant non-fat powdered milk, 3 tablespoons + 1 cup water = 1 cup non-fat milk

Skimmed, canned, 1 cup = 5 cups, whipped

PROTEIN

CHEESE

Cottage cheese, 1/2 pound = 1 cup

Cheese, grated, 1/4 pound = 1 cup

EGGS AND EGG SUBSTITUTES

Egg, raw, whole, 6 medium = 1 cup

Eggs, raw, in shell, 10 medium = 1 pound

Egg whites, 1 medium = 1-1/2 tablespoons

Egg whites, 9 medium = 1 cup

Egg yolks, 1 medium = 1 tablespoon

Egg yolks, 16 medium = 1 cup

Egg, hard-cooked, 1 = 1/3 cup, finely chopped

Egg substitute, liquid, 1/4 cup = 1 egg (see label)

Egg substitute, dry, 3 tablespoons = 1 egg (see label)

SEAFOOD AND FISH

Crab, fresh or frozen, cooked or canned, 1/2 pound (5-1/2- to 7-1/2- ounce tin) = 1 cup

Escargots, 9 snails = 1-1/2 ounces

Lobster, fresh or frozen, cooked, 1/2 pound = 1 cup

Oysters, raw, 1/2 pound = 1 cup

Scallops, fresh or frozen, shucked, 1/2 pound = 1 cup

Shrimp, cooked, 1 pound = 3 cups

Tuna, drained, canned, 6-1/2 to 7 ounces = 3/4 cup

STOCK BASE AND BOUILLON CUBES

BEEF STOCK BASE, POWDERED:

1 teaspoon = 1 bouillon cube

4 teaspoons + 1-1/4 cups water = 1 10-1/2-ounce can bouillon, undiluted

1 teaspoon + 5 ounces water = 5 ounces stock

1 teaspoon + 1 cup water = 1 cup bouillon

CHICKEN STOCK BASE, POWDERED:

1 teaspoon = 1 bouillon cube

1 teaspoon + 5 ounces water = 5 ounces stock

1 teaspoon + 1 cup water = 1 cup bouillon

VEGETABLES (DRIED)

Garbanzo beans, 1 pound, 2 cups = 6 cups, cooked

Kidney beans, 1 pound, 1-1/2 cups = 9 cups, cooked

Lima or navy beans, 1 pound, 2-1/2 cups = 6 cups, cooked

Rice, 1 pound, 2-1/2 cups = 8 cups, cooked

Split peas, 1 pound, 2 cups = 5 cups, cooked

VEGETABLES (FRESH)

Artichokes, 1/2 pound = 1 average

Asparagus, 1 pound, 18 spears = 2 cups, cut in 1-inch pieces

Avocado, 1 medium = 2 cups, chopped

Beans, green, 1 pound = 3 cups, chopped and cooked

Beets, 1 pound, medium-size = 2 cups, cooked and sliced

Bell pepper, 1/2 pound, 1 large = 1 cup, seeded and finely chopped

Broccoli, 1 pound, 2 stalks = 6 cups, chopped and cooked

Brussels sprouts, 1 pound, 28 average = 4 cups

Cabbage, 1 pound = 4 cups, shredded; 2-1/2 cups, cooked

Carrots, 1 pound, 8 small = 4 cups, chopped

Cauliflower, 1-1/2 pounds, 1 average = 6 cups, chopped and cooked

Celery, 1 stalk = 1/2 cup, finely chopped

Celery root, 1-3/4 pounds, 1 average = 4 cups raw, grated; 2 cups, cooked and mashed

Corn, 6 ears = 1-1/2 cups, cut

Cucumber, 1 medium = 1-1/2 cups, sliced

Eggplant, 1 pound, 1 medium = 12 1/4-inch slices; 6 cups, cubed

Lettuce, 1 average head = 6 cups, bite-size pieces

Lima beans, baby, 1 pound = 2 cups

Mushrooms, fresh, 1/2 pound, 20 medium = 2 cups raw, sliced

Okra, 24 medium = 1/2 pound

Onion, 1 medium = 1 cup, finely chopped

Parsnips, 1 pound, 6 average = 4 cups, chopped

Peas, in pods, 1 pound = 1 cup, shelled and cooked

Pimiento, 1, 4-ounce jar = 1/2 cup, chopped

Potatoes, 1 pound, 4 medium = 2-1/2 cups, cooked and diced

Pumpkin, 3 pounds, 1 average piece = 4 cups, cooked and mashed

Rutabagas, 1-1/2 pounds, 3 small = 2 cups, cooked and mashed

Spinach, 1 pound = 3-1/2 cups, uncooked; 1 cup, cooked

Squash, acorn, 1-1/2 pounds, 1 average = 2 cups, cooked and mashed

Squash, banana, 3 pounds, 1 average piece = 4 cups, cooked and mashed

Squash, spaghetti, 1 medium = 4 cups, cooked

Squash, summer, 1 pound, 4 average = 1 cup, cooked

Squash, zucchini, 1 pound, 2 average = 1-1/4 cups, cooked and chopped; 3 cups raw, diced

Tomatoes, 1 pound, 3 medium = 1-1/4 cups, cooked and chopped

Turnips, white, 1 pound, 3 small = 2 cups, peeled and grated; 1-1/4 cups, cooked and mashed

MISCELLANEOUS

Chocolate, 1 square, 1 ounce = 4 tablespoons, grated

Gelatin, sheet, 4 sheets = 1 envelope

Gelatin, powdered, 1/4-ounce envelope = 1 scant tablespoon

Yeast, fresh, 1 package = 2 tablespoons

Yeast, dry, 1 envelope (to be reconstituted in 2 tablespoons water) = 1-3/4 tablespoons

METRIC WEIGHTS

FOR DRY MEASURE:

Convert known ounces into grams by multiplying by 28

Convert known pounds into kilograms by multiplying by .45

Convert known grams into ounces by multiplying by .035

Convert known kilograms into pounds by multiplying by 2.2

FOR LIQUID MEASURE:

Convert known ounces into milliliters by multiplying by 30

Convert known pints into liters by multiplying by .47

Convert known quarts into liters by multiplying by .95

Convert known gallons into liters by multiplying by 3.8

Convert known milliliters into ounces by multiplying by .034

BIBLIOGRAPHY

Anderson, James W., M.D. *Diabetes–A Practical New Guide to Healthy Living.* New York: Arco Publishing, Inc., 1981.

Brody, Jane E. *Jane Brody's Nutrition Book.* New York: W. W. Norton & Co., 1981.

Church, Helen Nichols, and Pennington, Jean A. T. *Bowes and Church's Food Values of Portions Commonly Used.* 13th rev. ed. New York: Harper & Row Publishers, Inc., 1980.

Goulart, Frances Sheridan. *The Vegetarian Weight Loss Cookbook.* New York: Simon & Schuster, 1982.

Jones, Jeanne. *The Calculating Cook.* 2d ed., rev. San Francisco: 101 Productions, 1977.

———. *Diet for a Happy Heart.* 2d ed., rev. San Francisco: 101 Productions, 1981.

———. *Fabulous Fiber Cookbook.* 2d ed., rev. San Francisco: 101 Productions, 1979.

———. *More Calculated Cooking.* San Francisco: 101 Productions, 1981.

———. *Secrets of Salt-Free Cooking.* San Francisco: 101 Productions, 1979.

Jones, Jeanne, and Kientzler, Karma. *Fitness First: A 14-Day Diet and Exercise Program.* San Francisco: 101 Productions, 1980.

Kraus, Barbara. *The Dictionary of Sodium, Fats, and Cholesterol.* New York: Grosset & Dunlap, Inc., 1974.

U.S. Department of Agriculture. "Composition of Foods: Raw, Processed, Prepared." *Revised U.S.D.A. Agricultural Handbook,* no. 8. 1975.

U.S. Department of Agriculture. "Nutritive Value of American Foods in Common Units." *U.S.D.A. Agricultural Handbook,* no. 456. 1975.

U.S. Department of Health, Education and Welfare. *Healthy People– The Surgeon General's Report on Health Promotion and Disease Prevention, Background Papers.* 1979.

U.S. Senate Select Committee on Nutrition and Human Needs. *Dietary Goals for the United States.* 2d ed. December, 1977.

Zukin, Jane. *Milk Free Diet Cookbook.* New York: Sterling Publishing Co., 1982.

Index

RECIPE INDEX

GRAINS
Lemon Onion Bulgur, 170
Lentils au Gratin, 148
Powerful Porridge, 174
Stuffed Tomato Bowls, 148
Tabbouli, 174
Wild Rice Pilat, 175

MEAT
Lamb Chops Dijon, 165
Teriyaki Steak, 166

NOODLE DISHES
Fettuccine Cacciatore, 163
Pasta Primavera, 171
Seafood Chow Mein, 160
Toasted Chow Mein Noodles, 172
Vegetarian Lasagna, 153

POTATOES
Overbaked Potatoes, 172
Stuffed Baked Potato, 173
Tofu Stuffed Spud, 151

POULTRY
Cashew Chicken Salad, 162
Coq au Vin, 162
Fettuccine Cacciatore, 163
Lemon Chicken in Envelopes, 164
Tostada, 165

SOUPS
Blueberry Soup, 136
Egg Flower Soup, 136
Gazpacho, 137
Sherried Consommé, 138
Stracciatelle alla Romana, 138

STOCKS AND
   STOCK-BASED SAUCES
Beef Stock, 121
Brown Sauce, 122
Defatted Drippings, 123
Skinny Gravy, 123
Vegetable Stock, 124

TOPPINGS
Breakfast Cheese, 132
Coconut Sauce, 125
Curried Yogurt Dressing, 128
Dill Sauce, 125
Jelled Milk, 133
Jones Apple Butter, 178
Jones Basic Dressing, 128
Jones Pineapple-Ginger Dressing, 129
Jones Tomato Dressing, 130
Low-Calorie Catsup, 130
Major Jones Chutney, 131
Marinara Sauce, 126
Mock Sour Cream, 133
Mustard Dip, 131
Non-Fat Yogurt, 135
Sauterne Sauce, 126
Tofu Dressing or Dip, 132
Whipped "Cream," 135
White Sauce, Basic, 126
White Sauce, Fat-Free, 127

VEGETABLES
Asparagus Vinaigrette, 142
Herbed Vegetable Medley, 143
Stuffed Tomato Bowls, 148
Tomato Provençal, 143

VEGETARIAN ENTRÉES
Blender Crêpes, 145
Crêpes Florentine, 144
East Indian Carrot Casserole, 146
Huevos Rancheros, 147
Lentils au Gratin, 148
Moussaka, 150
Palak Paneer, 149
Stuffed Tomato Bowls. 148
Tamale Pie, 152
Tofu Stuffed Spud, 151
Vegetarian Lasagna, 153
Vegetarian Quiche, 154
Vegetarian White Chili, 155